AF340663

Community Medicine

Organization and Application of Principles

by

Leon R. Lezer, M.D.

VANTAGE PRESS
New York   Washington   Atlanta   Hollywood

To Phyllis

Contents

Foreword

Part I

Preface   3

A Organization of a Department of Preventive
   Medicine   9

B Teaching and Research in the New Department   18

C Staffing   26

D Program and Philosophy of Comprehensive Care   51

Part II

Preface   71

A The Wider Role of the University   73

B Formation of the Vermont Consultation Program   82

C Interrelationships With Other Concerned Groups   105

D The Heart of the Consultation Program—Rural
   Medical Needs   111

E Role of Paramedical Personnel in Consultation
  Service: 130

    The Physician   130
    The Public Health Nurse   132
    The Health Educator   135
    The Nutritionist   137
    The Social Scientist   139
    The Medical Social Worker   148
    The Statistician   153
    Interdisciplinary Relationships   154
    Implications for Curricula in Graduate Schools   160

F Relationship of the Consulting University to a State
  Health Department   168

G The Medical Society, the University, and the
  Health Department   180

H Relationship to Medical Societies   183

Conclusion   199

Appendixes   209

Notes   229

Foreword

The manuscript for this book was written in draft form in 1960, based on experience in the development of a Department of Preventive Medicine at the University of Vermont, College of Medicine, in Burlington, Vermont, beginning in July 1954. The introduction to the book describes the several facets of the department (known as departments of community medicine, social medicine, and the like in medical schools today). Balanced programs in teaching, research and extension of medical care services through the consultative process to communities from the hub of a university were established.

Many, many people were most supportive of these endeavors—they are far too numerous to list here. However, four persons must be recognized for their support of a most significant dimension.

Dr. Carl Borgman, President of the University of Vermont at that time, extended his futuristic outlook into all spheres of university responsibility. His major contribution to the organization and development of the New England Higher Education Compact lent a rationale to my concept of the Regional Medical Needs Board of Maine, New Hampshire, and Vermont.

Dr. George A. Wolf, Jr., then Dean of the College of Medicine, provided a climate through his leadership of not just impressive development of new medical school buildings, but the essential development of ideas as to the useful role of medical schools beyond the medical education process. I quote from a private communication of April 17, 1971, to me from Dr. Wolf: "The Regional Medical Needs Board was about 15 years ahead of itself . . . and . . . had all the elements in my mind which one needs today to plan for the delivery of health care. It had appropriate leadership, involvement of the educational institutions and opportunities for operations research." Dr. William H. Luginbuhl, now Dean of the College of Medicine at the University of Vermont, in a private communication of April 20, 1971, to me supports Dr. Wolf's statement: "I feel that in some ways you were a prophet before your time during your years in Vermont. It would seem that many are now trying to do what you advocated then."

Dr. Daniel F. Hanley, Executive Director of the Maine Medical Association, contributed wise counsel and substantive assistance in arousing the interest of organized medicine in Maine, New Hampshire, and Vermont, and among the leading political figures, the Honorable Frank E. Coffin (former Member of Congress from Maine) gave much time and effort in attempts to provide meaningful legislation for the effective delivery of health care to the nation.

Dr. Dean Fisher, Commissioner of Health and Welfare, State of Maine, provided stimulus for state governmental concern in a partnership between state governments and the private sector.

There is a fifth person whose diligence, ability and sense of humor made heavy tasks much lighter. I speak of Mrs. Allace C. Schalk of Burlington, Vermont . . . my secretary and administrative assistant throughout the years 1954–1961.

I am grateful to Muriel McLatchie Miller and Mrs. E. Tagrin, who at the time of the draft were responsible for the Medical Art Department of The Massachusetts General Hospital in Boston. They are responsible for the drawings in the text.

Needless to say, were it not for the confidence and generosity of the Commonwealth Fund of New York, little would have been accomplished in this demonstration of medical school teaching in community medicine and in the extension of services toward improved delivery of medical care by a university complex.

However late in publication, the contents of this book are still timely and relevant. Would that publication had occurred 15 years ago! . . . truly prophetic then! Unlike the unfinished symphony, there can be no unfinished publication! Hopefully, the reader of this book will find application of principles of teaching medical students and others community medicine, roles of the several disciplines professionally essential to that task and to the involvement of the varied skills of the allied health professionals from within the university to its "community."

Leon R. Lezer, M.D., M.P.H.

Nassau Shores
Massapequa, L.I., New York

PART

I

Preface

There is a natural reluctance to write of one's experiences, particularly if there is some question as to general interest in these experiences. After five years of developing a department of preventive medicine for the College of Medicine at the University of Vermont, I concluded there were many in the field of public health and preventive medicine, concerned with medical care problems, who would be interested in the approach to the development of this department. It also became clear that those concerned with medical education might have some interest in the approach taken at Vermont for the teaching of preventive medicine throughout the four years. This teaching is based on experiences in a consultation program, and on the universally recognized need to fuse the teaching of curative and preventive medicine. It was only after a series of visits to various medical schools, schools of public health, schools of social work and to some departments of sociology that I was convinced that writing on this subject would be a worthwhile effort. These visits, in which there was opportunity to talk with many individuals of prominence in public health, preventive medicine, and medical education, established the fact that there was an approach in the development of the department at Vermont that is of general interest.

While there has been a considerable amount of reading in the preparation of this manuscript, the bibliography is not lengthy. It is not lengthy because, for the most part, the material presented here was accumulated over a period of five years from experiences, observations, minutes of staff meetings, and the like. Not a great deal of time has been spent in repeating that which I

feel has been presented adequately in various publications
. . . and sometimes several times over. The development of a
consultation program in regional medical needs, stemming from a
university, is simply logical endeavor in conjunction with the organization of a department of preventive medicine at a university
medical school.

The objectives are no different from those that obtain in any
academic institution, namely, teaching and research. The added
objective of consultation through an extension-type service relates
to teaching and to research, but simultaneously is a logical endeavor of universities. There are many faculty members who provide consultation service on an individual basis. The program at
Vermont was one that had been developed as a system that is not
dependent on an individual, or upon particular individuals, but
rather upon the availability of skills that normally are found in
universities. If the ideas and actions cited here are useful to
others, I assume nevertheless that modifications would take place
depending upon the local setting.

Perhaps to the fickle finger of fate goes the credit for the
challenge and the opportunity which I had to return to my home
state in order to develop this program. The narrative gives the
sequence of events leading to an interest in rural medical care.
With the development of a facility in the rural area of my experience, in practice, it seemed logical that the state medical school
should take an active interest in this endeavor. With this premise
came the reason for visiting the dean of the medical school,
George A. Wolf, Jr. Dean Wolf was very much interested in
comprehensive medical care programs, and offered me an appointment to develop a department of preventive medicine along
the lines that I felt would be suitable for this particular school.

It was an interesting appointment in that the initial title was
Director of Health Studies. It was very astute to apply this title
in that it referred administratively to the office of the dean, and
provided opportunity for the necessary exploration in order to
develop a department.

As a result of visiting various professional schools, I know
that this study is potentially interesting to medical and public
health personnel and to the allied medical professions. To write a
book for the sake of writing a book is usually no author's purpose.
The principal objective in the writing of this book is to share with

others experiences which may be of value in the promotion of improved medical care and public health systems, including the frustrating, yet challenging and stimulating experiences of promoting new and amended legislation to better serve its purposes and intents.

The hypotheses that were set forth after a period of deliberation and planning for a program in preventive medicine that would be best suited to the University of Vermont, College of Medicine, were as follows:

A. *New England Board of Higher Education*
   Hypotheses:
   1. The New England Higher Education Compact in the field of medicine is particularly applicable to Maine, New Hampshire and Vermont, since Vermont has the only four-year medical school in these three states.
   2. Since the College of Medicine of the University of Vermont now provides many physicians for Maine, New Hampshire and Vermont, it is reasonable to concentrate on these three states in planning regional medical care as an extension of the Higher Education Compact.
   3. Maine, New Hampshire and Vermont have much in common from the standpoint of demography, political units, and socioeconomic situations which tend to make these three states a homogeneous region within which to study problems and plan solutions to those problems, particularly in the field of rural medical care.
   4. A clear understanding of medical care problems is necessary at the community level in the areas, presumably provided physicians by the University of Vermont, College of Medicine, and to which hopefully an increasing number of graduates will go, especially as general physicians.
   5. Research into requirements for physicians, nurses and other medical needs, particularly in rural areas of the three states, is a natural extension of the New England Board of Higher Education Compact.

B. *Organization of a Department of Preventive Medicine*
   Hypotheses:
   1. The University of Vermont, College of Medicine, is in

need of an organized department of preventive medicine functionally integrated into the teaching program at the bedside and ambulatory care level, as well as into the preclinical years.

2. To establish such a department in expectation of optimum gain to the student in concepts of total patient care, it is essential that there be a continuity of educational process extending from the liberal arts college through the four years of medical school. This necessitates two-way teaching and demonstration between the faculties of the liberal arts college and the college of medicine as well as opportunity for medical students to continue to participate in the liberal arts with special reference to sociology, anthropology and political science.

3. The preceding hypothesis is particularly practical at the University of Vermont because of the physical proximity of the liberal arts college and the College of Medicine on one campus.

4. The personnel of the department of preventive medicine should include a bio-statistician, a medical social worker, a public health nurse, a health educator, and a sociologist, with appropriate academic rating on the College of Medicine faculty. Such a team is essential not only for adequate teaching but also for planning and implementing medical care. Because of the working relationship to be established with the health departments of the three states, there will not be need for such personnel as epidemiologists, sanitarians, or nutritionists. These latter disciplines will be adequate on a part-time basis for an indefinite period. On the other hand, the work load in the department of preventive medicine will be too heavy to attempt part-time availability of those personnel listed above as faculty members needed on a full-time basis. The commissioners of health in the three states had already agreed to this working relationship.

5. The department of preventive medicine should be the focus within the College of Medicine for a home care program, ambulatory patient care and follow-up on any regional medical care implemented.

C. *Regional Medical Care Planning*
   Hypotheses:

1. As stated by hypotheses under Section II, Maine, New Hampshire, and Vermont constitute a natural region for the development of medical care planning as an extension of the New

England Higher Education Compact with the University of Vermont, College of Medicine, as the focus of activity.

2. The commissioners of health and the presidents of the medical societies of each of the states must first agree that such exploration, planning and implementation of a regional medical care program are the legitimate and logical functions of the University of Vermont, College of Medicine. There must be further agreement substantiated by a clear expression of interest in supporting such exploration, planning and implementation by joint conference of the two groups at the College of Medicine.

3. Dartmouth Medical School (two years)* and the Mary Hitchcock Hospital in Hanover, New Hampshire, must also accept the project. Furthermore, there must be consideration of ways and means in which the resources of these two institutions can properly be utilized and integrated in a regional medical care program.

4. The medical resources in Burlington must be assessed, and an evaluation made of medical needs to assure effort to:

a. Increase the scope of total patient care;
b. Provide comprehensive medical care in which adequate medical education can develop; and
c. Establish a base of operations that can function effectively as the focus of a regional medical care plan.

5. Costly field surveys are not indicated in exploring needs since (1) a vast amount of data is available to determine general needs as to availability of physicians and paramedical personnel, demography of areas and medical facilities; (2) cooperation of the state health departments and medical societies provide information that is current.

6. The New England Higher Education Compact, the organization of a department of preventive medicine and regional medical care planning are interrelated aspects of the objective, namely: The University of Vermont, College of Medicine, should serve as the focus of planning activity to meet medical care problems, particularly in the rural areas of Maine, New Hampshire, and Vermont.

*Now four years.

The development of a department of preventive medicine, embodying the principles set forth under these hypotheses, is described in the text of this book, dealing first with the development of a regional consultation program, and then, with the intramural activities of a department of preventive medicine including the roles of various personnel.

An intensive experience over a period of five years led to some impressions and to some conclusions as to the needs of medical education for the future. Consequently, I have been so audacious as to present, by skirmish only, some thoughts as to the process of medical education of the future, and some thoughts pertaining to development of programs of the future for the appropriate training of paramedical and social sciences personnel.

A

Organization of a
Department of Preventive Medicine

The past! the infinite greatness of the past! For what is the present after all, but a growth out of the past?
E. M. Forster, *A Passage to India*

To organize a department of preventive medicine was to draw upon the experiences of medical schools in the teaching of public health and preventive medicine. Particularly important were current trends in many medical schools in the reorganization of departments of preventive medicine, and in fact in the reorganization of medical school curricula as a whole. Teaching needs to be organized in such a way as to use the full significance of past experience for the present, but in such a way as to project principles into future application.

Today's student is heavily engrossed in current problems in medicine, but needs also to be given a framework of reference during his formal education for the sustained application of principles in his future practice—of continuing study as well as of a body of knowledge. In preventive medicine it is particularly important, because of changes in the economic and social order that lead to changes in the provision of medical services to the public. Cholecystitis is cholecystitis wherever it may be encountered, and coronary artery disease is coronary artery disease wherever today's student may be practicing tomorrow, but socioeconomic and demographic factors will be shifting. The student should gain from preventive medicine an understanding of the importance of the environmental factors, and of their relationship to biological factors that affect both physician and patient.

The foundation of sound medical practice is prevention of disease, early diagnosis, and prompt treatment. Through the implementation of this philosophy comes incidentally the most enduring doctor-patient relationship. The primary professional purpose of every physician should be to maintain health. Intermittent and episodic responsibility for a patient must give way to attitudes and concepts prompted by a challenging desire on the part of physicians to maintain health as well as to resolve pathology. The criteria for good health as defined by the World Health Organization—a state of complete physical, mental, and social well-being—must become the daily challenge of every physician. Physicians must be trained and equipped to prevent deterioration in sound health as well as to reverse the physiopathological conditions that will always beset the human organism in its struggle for environmental adaptation.

Certainly the physician's office, whether it is a private practice, a group practice, or an institutional practice, should be the center for efforts to meet this goal. It has been stated (Bean, 1954)[1] that leadership in clinical medicine has passed from the hands of the practicing physician into the ivory tower of our medical colleges, hospitals, and research institutes. Leadership in preventive measures for the maintenance of good health is the beginning of sound clinical medicine, and perhaps the physician in his office may find the opportunity to wrest the leadership in clinical medicine from the "ivory tower." Profiles of American medical practice indicate that the physician is not adequately oriented to the healthy organism in the conspicuous absence of visits to the physicians' offices for health evaluation. (Wells, 1956)[2].

The cornerstone of health evaluation is the physician's office. Orientation of the medical student to his future responsibility is therefore the beginning point. Here is the opportunity to develop an orientation to, and a sustained interest in, the *healthy* person. So long as our medical schools emphasize primarily, and almost exclusively, the physician's responsibility for resolution of organic pathology, he will not be particularly keen about taking the necessary time to conduct a thorough examination in the absence of a presenting complaint. In this era of marked changes—almost revolutionary in concept and in nature—in medical schools, there is beginning to be increased emphasis on the changing role of the physician in meeting a changing demand for medical care. It is not without cause that many persons hesitate "to bother" their physicians with a request for examination in the absence of organic symptomatology. And neither is it without basis to say that this hesitancy stems at least in part from the physician's attitude.

Efforts are being made to achieve a better understanding of the ecology of the medical student as well as of the etiology of disease. Professor E. Lowell Kelly, Chairman of the Psychology Department of the University of Michigan, has conducted a series of motivation tests on groups of medical students and residents. He was searching for the answer to the question, What kinds of people are going into medicine today? His impressions are not heartening (Kelly, 1957)[3]. It is a little startling to learn that his studies justify the conclusion that many medical students, if they were not seeking to become physicians, would become manufacturers, businessmen, production managers, or engineers. They would not become teachers, clergymen, social workers—that is, professionals interested in serving the welfare of mankind. This is not to suggest that all of today's physicians are not the type of person Professor Kelly was searching for in his analysis of present-day students. Far from it. But it does call attention to the need for awareness on the part of medical educators that the orientation of the candidate for medical practice will determine whether the public receives partial or total medical care, maintenance of health as well as the resolution of organic pathology.

The whole matter of medical education as it relates to physicians' attitudes, and in turn to their influence on patients and families and communities in assuming responsibility for complete health maintenance, is currently under searching analysis. It is mentioned here because of its important relationship to the philosophy and objectives of a department of preventive medicine. Programs fusing preventive and curative medicine that have clinical appeal to students must be developed. This was an essential tenet in the philosophy that shaped the development of the new department of preventive medicine at the University of Vermont.

When I accepted responsibility for the organization of a department of preventive medicine at the University of Vermont, College of Medicine, I did so with the important condition that I would not have any immediate responsibility either for teaching, or for introducing new elements of teaching, in preventive medicine. Thus I had time to become familiar with existing methods of teaching public health and preventive medicine and with the current status at the college of medicine.

I asked to meet with senior medical students in groups of four or five for four to five consecutive hours. These sessions continue and are known as conferences in preventive medicine. Initially, the major purpose of these conferences was to obtain from the students their concepts of preventive medicine as related to the private practice of medicine. While some newer concepts in preventive medicine were discussed, the sessions served me more than they did the student by giving me some insight into the students' strengths and weaknesses in preventive medicine. It was quite obvious that previous students' success in meeting the requirements in public health and preventive medicine in medical school and National Board examinations had resulted largely from "cramming" rather than from a working knowledge or a full appreciation of the fusion of preventive and curative medicine in practice.

Several premises shaped the approach that was taken in the development of the department:

1. It would be futile for one to list simply the number of hours that one would like to have available for the teaching of preventive medicine in any of the four years.

2. At Vermont newer concepts of preventive medicine teaching, and the experimentation in teaching that was taking place across the country, were conspicuous by their absence. These concepts must be introduced to members of the Curriculum Committee before any specific requests for curriculum time were made.

3. While the teaching of prevention in medicine should be a concern of every clinical department, there should be an administrative focus of emphasis in teaching preventive medicine. Otherwise, that which is "everybody's business soon becomes nobody's business." Furthermore, the number of staff to be involved,

budgetary considerations, and research programs required that there be a separate, departmental entity in order to establish, maintain, and increase the impact of preventive medicine on the total medical school curriculum.

4. Since preventive medicine, when properly applied, is both a basic and a clinical science, it is important to establish preventive medicine teaching in the first year of medical school and to maintain a thread of progressive continuity throughout the four years. Teaching of preventive medicine will then be much more effective in a sustained fusion of cure and prevention.

5. If one is gradually to develop acceptable attitudes toward a methodology and subject matter that are not traditionally included in the medical student's concept of the practice of medicine, it is important to establish contact with the medical student when he enters medical school and to maintain it throughout the four years. Otherwise the medical student views teaching in preventive medicine as an interference with, or at best extraneous to, his preoccupation with diagnosis and treatment.

6. Opportunities for preventive medicine teaching in collaboration with other departments should be evaluated. Conversely, the concepts of preventive medicine should be more consistently included in the daily teaching of other clinical departments.

7. In view of the department's proposed emphasis on meeting medical needs in a predominately rural region, it was important that some aspect of the medical school training equip graduates for practice in rural situations. The opportunity for developing this kind of teaching eventually came through the then existing "city service" program. The reorganization of this service into a general practice demonstration unit with teaching of comprehensive medical care is discussed later. If emphasis were placed on the social as well as the clinical aspects of preventive medicine in the first two years, students presumably would be better attuned to the social aspects of medicine in such a unit. This approach in preventive medicine would, however, have to be deferred until the faculty became more familiar with the general philosophy behind preventive medicine teaching. Furthermore, acquisition of personnel and the development of a rural consultation program necessarily took precedence over the development of such a unit.

8. Newer concepts of public health and preventive medicine were paramount in the thinking and planning of medical educators and medical administrators all over the country, and volumes of material on the subject were available. The thinking of prominent men and women had been recorded, discussed and debated in the literature, at scientific assemblies, and in the press. All that remained to be accomplished was the adaptation of an acceptable philosophy in the teaching of preventive medicine to the local situation. The acceptable philosophy had to be weighed in terms of local needs, culture, and economic capacity to proceed with implementation. The point of reference in planning had to be, as always, measurement of the status quo.

9. An inventory of facilities, personnel, attitudes, fears, hopes, and ambitions had to be made. Search for restlessness or intellectual curiosity about the future, readily apparent in a few instances, was indicated. Evaluation of the local situation proceeded, but had to be geared to what could be done by only one person over a period of time limited enough that momentum toward accomplishment of the goal would not be lost. The evaluation therefore was superficial, but did at least serve to suggest a course of action leading toward the objectives. Needless to say, the evaluation has continued.

10. It was obvious that preventive medicine as a unit of teaching in the medical school curriculum required an entire reorganization. Little of the curriculum could be retained in its present structure if the level of advancement of most medical schools was to be equaled. Thus, planning could be wholly free, rather than limited by the need to restructure a preexisting program. This was fortunate, for it greatly facilitated accomplishment of the two objectives within one department: development of a consultation program on regional medical needs, and organization of a new academic department.

The haunting question was: What kind of a department of preventive medicine should this one be? Certainly it would have much in common with departments in other medical schools. But it had also to be organized in such a way as to assure the teaching of total patient care with its strength of action based on system of organization and function rather than on specific individuals. It must be a department balanced between public health, environmental medicine, and medical care problems.

In the study of the medical care facilities, the information was obtained on the following areas:

1. Administrative organization
2. Philosophy of the administration as to purpose and obligations
3. Financial aspects—charges, costs, methods of collection, sources of income
4. Departmental data
    a. Philosophy of department head
    b. Attitude toward other departments
    c. Attitude toward economic groups
    d. Interdepartmental relationships
    e. Understanding of budget operation
    f. Observation of attitude toward patients, physicians, nurses, and students
5. Teaching values
    a. Student-patient time relationship
    b. Instructor-student time relationship
    c. Number of clinics
    d. Type of clinics
    e. Number of patients per student
    f. Methods of clinical teaching
    g. Responsibilities of students
    h. Continuity of student-patient relationship
6. Records: Inpatient and Outpatient
    a. Completeness
    b. Student comments
    c. Evidence of total evaluation of patient, individual, medical, social, and economic factors
    d. Evidence of continuity of care
    e. Follow-up interest
    f. Interdepartmental referral
    g. Relationship to referring physician
    h. Relationship to community, home, and family

As Director of Health Studies as well as Assistant Professor of Preventive Medicine, I enjoyed an administrative relationship with the dean's office that provided the organizational base for the exploration of departmental and interdepartmental interests in the development of a teaching program in preventive medicine. Aside from information being obtained from this study of potentials for the teaching of preventive medicine, reports were submitted to the hospitals concerned. As requested by the administrators, the reports contained important recommendations concerning university–teaching hospital relationships, especially with respect to responsibility in the health field and resulting financial obligations. At this early date a study of the then existing "dispensary and city service" program was made and plans developed for its reorganization. Following release of the report to the administration of the hospitals, considerable time was spent in advising on implementation of some of the recommendations, especially those concerned with clinic operation and medical records.

A department of preventive medicine must work closely with community agencies if it is effectively to emphasize environmental medicine. Therefore, concurrently with the study of local medical care facilities, voluntary and official agencies were visited. In each instance, there was a discussion of ideas relating to a department of preventive medicine, the importance of the agency to teaching and its possible role in teaching, the agency's interest in participating in the program, and the college's potential role in supporting the agency's program.

The agency's organization was also discussed, including the origin of administrative organization, its geographic area of operation, functions, budget, size and professional qualifications of its staff, patient load and types of cases, educational program, and its problems and future plans.

Interagency relationships were explored, and information sought on the agency's previous experience with the medical school.

The immediate value of these interviews was that:

1. Communication had been established between available voluntary agencies and a department of preventive medicine.

2. Interest in a new program at the College of Medicine was created.

3. Expression of a desire to be affiliated on an organized teaching basis was obtained.

4. Joint interest between the medical school and community agencies in promoting total patient care at the community level had been aroused.

A variety of official public agencies were also visited, and mutual objectives similar to those with voluntary agencies established.

Demonstration of total patient care through cooperative action is much more meaningful to the student than lectures about it. While efforts to achieve comprehensive medical care teaching within the department of preventive medicine were consonant with current and popular endeavors to apply the tools of preventive medicine to total patient care, a major motive was to give medical students a genuine opportunity to compare the practice of general medicine with the practice of other specialties. This, it was recognized, would require the participation of general physicians in the program when the time came to reorganize the "city service" and dispensary program. Without their participation there could be no real demonstration of comprehensive medical care through general medical practice and, consequently, no demonstration of the fact that the first line of defense in preventive medicine is the major responsibility of the family physician.

B

Teaching and Research
in the New Department

The organization of a new department, or rather the reorganization of public health teaching into a department of preventive medicine, immediately poses a problem of curriculum time. Berry (1953)[4] reminds us that the word curriculum means "a running" or a "race course," and further cites the problem of the "massive medical curriculum which has grown more by accretion than by design." In organizing the Department of Preventive Medicine, effort was focused on providing the student with pertinent information in the field of preventive medicine, and incidentally to equip him to pass medical school and licensure examinations successfully. The department was designed to equip the physician of tomorrow so that he would be able to apply principles in remaining abreast of important changes in the field and to remain aware of socioeconomic changes, with particular reference to gaps in the availability of medical technology and delivery of medical care. As Ogburn (1922) pointed out, ". . . scientific advances are great and social adjustments are slow."

The preventive medicine program reached the medical student in each of his four years of study. For administrative purposes, the department was divided into four divisions: the General Division, which included a regional consultation program; the Division of General Medicine; the Division of Rehabilitation; and the Division of Occupational Medicine.

The Division of General Medicine covered the general practice demonstration unit and the comprehensive medical care demonstration known as the Family Care Unit. The Division of Rehabilitation was organized in the second year of the program.

Teaching in Rehabilitation consisted of several hours integrated into the courses of the departments of anatomy, physiology, medicine, surgery, and pediatrics. Teaching in Rehabilitation therefore reached medical students in all four years. Teaching was by lecture, seminar and/or demonstration, and covered electrical stimulation to motor points, gerontology and geriatrics, cardiac work classification, speech pathology, electrodiagnostic techniques, and electrophysiology.

The Division of Occupational Medicine remained weak, and the teaching of occupational and industrial medicine left much to be desired. There was an opportunity to strengthen the program through arrangements with local industry. The program in occupational medicine was confined to self-study assignments for students in the second year, and two fellowships at a local industrial plant for third-year students. Because the graduates of the school were dispersed about the country, and would be concerned with problems in occupational medicine to varying degrees, it was important that this deficit in teaching be corrected, and plans were made toward this end.

In the first year approximately seventeen hours were devoted to the teaching of human ecology (Lezer, 1951)[5].

Demography has become the core of problems in the medical as well as in the economic and social fields. Greater population growth and movement coupled with a proportionate increase in the number of the very young, as well as longevity, have forced a focus upon total environmental factors affecting the human organism.

There is a growing awareness of the need to call upon the social and behavioral sciences to comprehend fully the impact of environmental factors affecting man's health and therefore his relationship to society. Increasingly, attention is being focused upon the natural history of disease—and upon the natural history of health. This cannot be complete without sociological definition and interpretation. The plea at mid-century is to include the assessment of the status of man in his environment without excluding the strictly biological approach. The theory of multiple causation of disease cannot be fully sustained without full exploration of social as well as clinical epidemiology. Increasing exposure to long-term illness, degenerative disease, mental illness, and accidents makes the time opportune for an effective holistic approach to medical practice and medical research.

Human ecology, then, must become a part of the deliberate approach to the practice of medicine. The teaching of human ecology can serve as one of the tools in medical education for making the future physician aware of the importance of fully understanding his patient, the biological unit in which he lives, and the environmental forces acting upon both. In effect, it may serve to focus attention upon the patient and his family, as was the custom of "the old family physician." With the highest regard and respect for the much eulogized family physician of the past, one must remember that the lack of tools at his command necessitated long periods of time with the patient and his family. Some mechanism must be employed in order to reestablish the intimate relationship between physician and patient without loss of expediency through the use of rapid means of diagnosis, therapy, and delegation of responsibility to myriads of personnel in the modern structure of medical care.

For some time prior to coming to the University of Vermont, the author had an opportunity to work closely with graduates of medical schools in two large metropolitan hospitals. During this time, considerable thought had been given to the need for some mechanism in the medical school curriculum which would provide the student with broader understanding of his patient as a member of society, as well as an intricate understanding of the disease process which overtakes the patient. The development of a department of preventive medicine at the University of Vermont provided the opportunity to explore possibilities. Through the teaching of human ecology and the availability of a sociologist, a health educator, and a medical social worker on the faculty, different points of view could be coupled with those of physicians in teaching this subject matter.

The first year of medicine was chosen for several reasons:

1. It seemed important to begin the teaching of preventive medicine as such early in the curriculum and to continue contact with students throughout the four years. Hopefully, such continuity would lead to student understanding of the need to fuse preventive philosophy and techniques with curative procedures.

2. Since human ecology would naturally stress the importance of understanding the function of the individual as a whole in relation to environmental forces, it seemed important to attempt this while the student is of necessity studying details of structure and function. This timing would serve to preclude focusing attention only on the parts in structure and function and would inculcate from the early days of medical school the need to understand the whole in relation to external forces and conditions as well as the relationship of the parts to the whole.

3. Since the student at Vermont concentrates heavily in anatomy and since the cadaver is the physical body that housed the individual, it seemed clear that utilization of the cadaver history might possibly leave some lasting effect on the student as to the importance of the intangibles as well as the tangibles in medicine.

4. Some time and effort had already been given to the establishment of a pilot program in combining liberal education with medical education in Vermont.

There was some concern that use of the cadaver history might be emotionally traumatic to the medical student. Psychiatrically, there was valid criticism concerning such a possibility. It did not seem reasonable that a student might be emotionally traumatized when reading something of the life of an individual whose body he was systematically "destroying." The first year, therefore, only half the class had available to them the life histories of the cadavers. Since that first year, however, the entire class has had cadaver histories for teaching purposes in human ecology.

The life history of an individual presents a complete profile from which retrospective conclusions may be drawn. Not unlike interpretation of the signs observed by the pathologist at autopsy are the signs of events in an individual's life which may serve as useful indications of differences in life patterns. There are also indications of points at which the physician could have served as instigator of change in social forces as well as in physiological ones. In other words, the life history of the cadaver might be plotted in the same way as the biological gradient for a particular disease.

Methodology

Because of the problem of curriculum time noted above, and with the desire to combine ecology with anatomy, the cooperation of the Department of Anatomy was obtained. Time was arranged for students to attend a series of seven orientation lectures in human ecology followed by seminars in which the life history of the cadaver was discussed. Since the first year (1955), human ecology has been taught in alternate weeks with psychobiology. The Dean's Conference time has been allocated for this purpose. Following the orientation lectures given by the sociologist, the students meet in seminar for two 2-hour periods on alternate weeks. During these seminar periods, the cadaver history obtained by the medical social worker the previous summer is discussed with emphasis on social, cultural, and economic factors in the life of the individual as they related to medical care problems. Participating in this seminar are the physician (including the professor of anatomy and/or his associates), the medical sociologist, the health educator, and the medical social worker. During 1958 a public health nurse, who is also full-time on the faculty in preventive medicine, was added to the group.

Periodically throughout the year additional lectures are given according to need as revealed through seminar discussions. Again the anatomy department has cooperated fully in providing seven additional lecture hours throughout the year for this purpose.

In the case histories utilized in the seminars on human ecology, emphasis is placed on the social and economic factors. While the students are much interested in the clinical aspects, the seminar is designed to suit the level of their medical training. Students identify ecological factors in health and in disease which would have been promoted or avoided by a physician keenly aware of his responsibilities for comprehensive medical care. The seminars provide an opportunity, too, to introduce the student to various social and legislative problems, and to concepts of agency responsibility, both voluntary and official, in the total care of the patient. The case history is authentic, only the real name of the patient being replaced with another of the same ethnic derivation. The social worker had additional case history material if it were requested, or needed, in the seminar.

At the end of the year, the students had an exercise in human ecology which usually involves a case comparable to the case histories used in the seminar. The students wrote a discussion of the case, identifying factors of ecological importance in the discharge of the physician's responsibility to the patient, to the family, and to the community. Further experimentation with this course may result in modification, but the cadaver history will almost certainly still be used. This technique can contribute importantly to the development of concepts of the whole problem while the student is being given detailed training focused on the structural and functional aspects.

The teaching staff in the seminar included the physician, the medical social worker, and the sociologist. The objectives of the teaching program in human ecology were met adequately by this faculty.

In the second year, twelve hours were devoted to applied medical statistics (vital statistics and biometrics). The course was designed to introduce some of the concepts used in medical statistics as well as some of the general methods of statistical analysis to the medical students. Both vital statistics and biometrics are covered. In general, the purpose of the course was to give students a "working knowledge" of statistics that would aid them in interpreting and understanding the statistics they encounter in the course of their medical education and postgraduate education, and in their later reading of current literature.

In the second year the students received five hours of introduction to clinical epidemiology during which the basic and newer concepts in epidemiology, particularly as they apply to noncommunicable disease, chronic disease, accident prevention, and mental illness, were presented in summary form. Reference was constantly made to the "old tools" of preventive medicine so that the student would perceive the application of constructive epidemiology to current and future medical care problems. The hours in clinical epidemiology were increased in order that there would be more opportunity for laboratory exercises in clinical epidemiology and increased use of applied medical statistics.

Only five hours was given to the teaching of medical care systems. A brief survey of the organization and structure of medical care programs in the United States was presented and some approaches of other countries to the problems of delivery of medical care were introduced. The relationship of federal, state, and local health agencies to the practice of medicine was described. In general, an effort was made to give the student some orientation to specific institutions with which he would be associated during clinical clerkships and later medical career.

In order to introduce applied medical statistics, clinical epidemiology, and medical care in the second year, the thirty hours that had been devoted to public health and preventive medicine teaching were revised. A self-study program was initiated for the second year students which removes from lecture hours a body of material which the student can easily read by himself. The readings cover sanitation, communicable diseases and some of the arthropod-borne diseases, and occupational and industrial medicine. During the semester four free periods were assigned, replacing lecture hours, in order that the student could have this time for the assigned material. Subject matter was assigned to groups of two to four students. An advisor was available if the students wished to discuss any of the subject matter. At the end of the year each group submitted a brief typewritten report on the subject assigned. These typewritten reports were compiled into a manual of "Notes in Public Health" and returned to the class the following year. Four hours were reserved during which the groups of students reported to the entire class.

By the beginning of the third year (or the end of the second year) there were usually five to eight students with fellowships in preventive medicine and public health. The fellowships had been granted largely by the National Foundation, which is no longer providing such assistance. During the summer, the fellows on a project worked under the supervision of assigned faculty members, and at the end of the summer, each wrote a report on his particular assignment presenting recommendations and conclusions, if they were in order. Encouragement and guidance were given to the end that these reports might be submitted for publication.

Preventive medicine teaching in the third and fourth years consisted primarily of a comprehensive medical care experience in a home care visiting program.

During the fourth year there were eight one-hour conferences on preventive medicine, in which six to eight seniors participated on a rotating basis. Although these conferences were used in the past to discuss newer and basic concepts of preventive medicine, and to elicit the student's level of understanding of preventive medicine today and its possibilities for the future, they became clinical, preventive medicine conferences. The conferences continued to provide the opportunity for small group discussion of the important implications of preventive medicine for the student's future practice of medicine regardless of his field of endeavor.

During the fourth year there were eight hours of gerontology conferences for groups of five and six students. The medical social worker had a major responsibility for these conferences, which took place in cooperation with the DeGoesbriand Memorial Hospital and a home for the aged affiliated with the hospital. Each student was responsible for a comprehensive evaluation of one elderly resident of the home. The evaluation was then discussed by the student group under the leadership of a clinician especially interested in problems of the aging, and with the participation of a physician responsible for the continuity of patient care and a social worker. Students were helped to understand the differences in the physiology, symptomatology, emotional patterns and social problems of the aged, and how the physician can better deal with these differences and problems.

In the development of the Vermont program the teaching of comprehensive medical care received an emphasis commensurate with the importance it has assumed in the thoughts of all concerned with medical care today. The accent on an holistic philosophy of medical education is evolutionary in nature. As control has been established over communicable and infectious diseases, and as technological services have become increasingly available, there has been a natural turning of attention toward conditions which do not yet respond to present curative methods.

C

Staffing

Personnel

A major facet in the development of the Department of Preventive Medicine at the University of Vermont was exploring the use of paramedical and social science personnel on a full-time basis in a medical school setting.

The personnel selected to serve as full-time faculty members in the Department of Preventive Medicine represented professional fields considered by a growing number of educators to be important to the development of an holistic approach to the teaching of medicine, and whose potential contributions to a medical education program, including research, I particularly wanted to observe.

Appointments were made in sociology and in medical social service during the first year. The following year, a health educator, a statistician, a public health nurse, and a nutritionist were added. It soon became necessary to appoint a second full-time physician because of the development of the comprehensive medical care teaching program, and for the same reason, a second public health nurse and another medical social worker.

All of the personnel were appointed with the knowledge and understanding that they were participating in the organization and development of a department, a major emphasis of which was to be a regional consultation program in rural medical needs, and concurrently, in an examination of the potential roles of their various disciplines in a medical school. For some time research had to be confined to the studies pertaining to the development of the regional consultation program. In the third and fourth years of the program, however, it was possible to begin to branch out into other areas of research according to the interests of the person concerned and his ability to attract research funds.

At the peak of the department demonstration the full-time staff included two physicians, one health educator, two public health nurses, two medical social workers, one nutritionist, one statistician, and one sociologist.

In addition, eight general physicians with part-time appointments participated as clinical associates. The executive secretary who was with the department from the beginning of the development of the program became the administrative assistant. During the peak of the development of the program, there were seven secretaries in addition to the administrative assistant.

The full-time staff of the department consisted of: three physicians; one medical social worker; one public health nurse; one statistician; one administrative assistant; one statistical clerk; one staff nurse; one general office aide, and three secretaries.

Twelve physicians in general medicine, gerontology, public health, and rehabilitation, one sociologist, one anthropologist, one educator, and one specialist in speech rehabilitation also served on a part-time basis.

Because of the emphasis on exploration of the potential role of social science and paramedical personnel in medical school teaching, formal staff meetings were held regularly at least once each month, and informal meetings more frequently. All of the appointments were made with the understanding that they did not necessarily represent a conviction that there is in fact an appropriate place in the medical school structure for each of these disciplines, a procedure which caused a certain amount of frustration. Concern about status, and the opportunity to establish the importance of each of these disciplines inevitably arose. This concern applied not only to the individual, but also to success or failure that might reflect on the whole professional group he represented. The current state of uncertainty of various professional groups concerning their specific responsibilities in medical schools is at once intriguing and alarming. It is not yet clearly established how, and to what extent, each of these disciplines can, in its own unique way, contribute substance of importance to the future physician. And the contribution must be unique, since it would be pointless to increase either the cost of medical education or the complexity of the medical school curriculum by introducing a new discipline to present material already being offered although perhaps with a different terminology. The departments of medicine and pediatrics, for example, usually teach the relative importance of ethnicity and economics in certain disease patterns. Physicians teaching clinical epidemiology usually deal with demographic forces in the spread and control of disease, including noninfectious and noncummunicable diseases and conditions.

With a staff new to the medical school setting, whose specific preparation for medical school teaching was negligible, I had to be available to the staff for frequent meetings and informal sessions. In a sense, teaching at a residency level was required. At the same time, it was important that this not interfere with the staff's assumption of responsibility appropriate to the obligations imposed by academic rank. They had to be given freedom to develop their own ideas and concepts, even though these might be contrary to the judgment of the director or inconsistent with the utilitarian point of view on medical education. Each discipline had to be given scope for originality if some understanding of the potential role the newer, nonmedical professions might play in a medical school setting was to be achieved.

It was important that the intentions and goals of the program be made clear to the faculty of other departments of the medical school, both informally in personal discussions and formally in meetings with the curriculum committee. Thus, a climate of general understanding of the program's experimental approach was created and the faculty accepted the research goal of trying to determine the potentials of allied professional personnel in medical school teaching.

On the small campus of the University of Vermont, interest in the activities of the department as a whole extended to other colleges, notably to the College of Liberal Arts and to the College of Education. Later, this interest served as the basis for the development of intercollege participation in the teaching program. The fact that the program's sociologist was allowed to devote some time to teaching in the Department of Sociology was an important consideration in the development of this interest. The program faculty had previously participated in the program of the Department of Nursing in the College of Education.

The conclusions presented here on the functions, uses and training of this variety of personnel are based on six years of intensive work with personnel representing the various professional fields which, to one degree or another, are functioning in the medical education system. It is appropriate that the discussion begin with the physician who, presumably, is prepared for full-time teaching in preventive medicine.

The physician teaching preventive medicine must have as much zest for long-range satisfaction as he had in his earlier years for the immediate satisfaction of curing the ill, repairing the wounded, bringing new life into the world, and easing the pain of death for both patient and family. The physician in preventive medicine teaching must be convinced that actual fusion of preventive and curative medicine is practicable. He must believe that the student's charted course should be one that will help him to realize that the actual course he navigates in his education and later in his practice has many points apart from mere diagnosis and treatment. As a teacher of preventive medicine, he must feel, and arouse in his students, a more than perfunctory interest in the political, social, cultural, and scientific events which have led to current concepts of public health and preventive medicine.

Rosen (1958)[6] points out that "the provision of medical service is an activity involving interaction between two or more human beings, thus creating a social system. At the same time the participants in this system are also members of other larger and smaller social systems, which form the greater part of their environment, and which exert a determining influence on their thought and action." It is only with a full knowledge of this environment that physicians can appropriately take their places as teachers of preventive medicine. While a variety of physicians may assume responsibility for the academic direction of preventive medicine, the specifications for adequate performance in this field are just as important for the determination of competency as are the specifications for competent performance in other special fields. Because of the breadth and depth of the subject matter of preventive medicine, persons with a variety of backgrounds may attain academic positions in this field. There is no uniform requirement in our medical schools covering those who assume responsibility for the direction of departments of preventive medicine. An internist, for example, may function well as director of a department of preventive medicine. However, it is important that any internist directing a department of preventive medicine either be a veteran of additional training in the field of public health and preventive medicine, or surround himself with staff who have formal graduate training in preventive medicine and experience in one of the several fields that comprise preventive medicine.

Smillie (1955)[7] pointed out that the physician is beginning to realize that ". . . the practice of medicine encompasses a great deal more than direct physician-patient relationship. He must know his community resources that have been developed for prevention of illness as well as for social readjustment. He must work with health officials, district nurses, social service departments, Blue Cross, Blue Shield, and other devices for providing adequate financial support for medical care. He must be aware of a rehabilitation facility that is available in his community, and must himself be an active force in the community in promoting new facilities to provide for unmet needs." Dr. Smillie further pointed to the important function a department of preventive medicine can perform by serving as a liaison between the social forces of the community and the medical college with its ancillary hospitals and clinic services.

The physician directing the activities of a department of preventive medicine must be one who is not distressed by heavy administrative responsibilities. He should be sufficiently interested in medical care administration and social legislation so that he can impart with enthusiasm his convictions that the responsibility of the future physician lies not only in the dispensing of technological services, but also in the promotion of broader concepts for improved health and welfare services in his community, in his state, and indeed, in the nation as a whole. The attributes of the physician in a department of preventive medicine are essentially those that exemplify the ideals of comprehensive medical care. To be able to accept the participation of others, even if on an experimental basis, in a shared teaching responsibility, and to establish relationships which lead to the efficient integration of curative and preventive medicine through conjoint interdepartmental action, demands a working knowledge of the principles of public health practice.

The usual preparation of a physician in preventive medicine is through formal graduate training in a school of public health. By and large, schools of public health meet the technical requirements of preparation for teaching in preventive medicine. Added to technical subjects in the field of preventive medicine and public health, however, should be a period of training and experience in educational methods per se.

Paramedical Personnel and Social Science Personnel

A variety of personnel are being utilized, in one way or another, in medical schools with the alleged goal of teaching comprehensive medical care. That there is a need for some social science teaching is not denied. But the fact that this need exists raises serious questions as to the sophistication of the new college graduate. One should be able to assume that a liberal arts education would give all of these potential leaders some understanding of the social, economic, and cultural problems that at once benefit and harass the forward movement of civilization. Such is not the case. It is somewhat appalling to realize how many of our college graduates seem to have only a nodding acquaintance with the history of civilization, and of the cultural and economic forces affecting daily living. The deficiency in this area is apparently greater than the obvious deficiency in the ability to articulate, to express one's self clearly in writing, and to communicate intelligently with different levels of society. A graduate school, in this instance a college of medicine, is therefore forced to take these deficiencies into account, and to attempt to provide somewhere in an already crowded curriculum an orientation to the environmental factors that affect proficiency in the practice of medicine.

Stocking (1959)[8] makes an eloquent plea for support of the "humanities" as essential to the mature development of the educated individual. He decried the utilitarian bias which the country in general shows politically, educationally, and scientifically, but astutely pointed out that teachers of the liberal arts have so far failed effectively to state the case for more adequate support by convincingly elucidating the value of a liberal education for professional groups. Again, one must note that the ideal college preparation should not leave professional schools, including engineering, medicine, nursing, and law, wondering about how adequately prepared their students are for the most skillful application of their professional knowledge. These graduate schools are currently seeking supplementary training for their students in the very fields in which every college-educated person should have become competent merely in the course of a sound educational development. Until college students consistently receive a type of higher education that gives them full appreciation of the cultural, economic, and social factors operating in the civilization of which they are members, graduate schools such as the medical college must find ways and means of bridging this gap, possibly through radical changes in selection and in the continuity of professional and liberal education.

That a large number of patients do have social problems has been documented many times. In an evaluation of the teaching of social and environmental medicine, Curran and Cockerill (1948)[9] point out that in a study of more than 600 cases at the Massachusetts General Hospital, all but half a dozen of the patients had social problems related to illness. In most instances, there were three or four social problems complicating the illness. These social problems affecting recovery, if they were not also principal precipitating factors of illness, included financial difficulties, personality and attitudes, the costs of medical care, problems of convalescence, family relationships, occupational adjustments, and illness of other family members. Dr. G. Canby Robinson (1939)[10,11], in a study of an unselected series of patients admitted to the Johns Hopkins Dispensary, showed that adverse social conditions related to illness existed in 65 percent of the cases.

That medicine is a natural *and* social science is proclaimed by many. That it is first of all a biological science, and one which cannot be applied without sound preparation in the biological sciences, need not be forgotten when appropriate concepts of the social sciences are integrated with medical education.

In considering the potential contribution of paramedical and social science personnel to a medical education program, the following questions are pertinent:

1. What is the role of the social scientist or the paramedical person* in medical education?

2. How can allied professional groups contribute to the process of medical education?

3. What difference does it make if these particular disciplines are represented in medical education?

In other words, is there a unique contribution that a particular discipline can make to medical education that cannot be made by any other, particularly by those basic science and clinical fields that are now traditionally a part of medical education?

These were the questions before the full-time nonmedical staff as they considered how their particular skills might be applied in the medical education process. Coupled with the constant encouragement of self-criticism, they effectively precluded any premature or unfounded claim of unique responsibility by the staff. For example, social science concepts enter into the teaching of medicine, pediatrics, and, to some extent, surgery. Clinical epidemiology, by its very nature, takes into consideration the relativity of social, cultural, and economic factors. If the paramedical person or the social scientist is to bring something into the curriculum that would not otherwise be there, he cannot simply borrow subject matter that is already taught by clinicians or others. And, if all clinical departments placed reasonable emphasis upon the teaching of preventive factors in the practice of medicine, they would be covering much of the material that is important in the teaching of comprehensive medical care.

The participation of paramedical and social science personnel in medical school curricula demands a somewhat utilitarian approach. The training of a physician emphasizes the development of skills that will be of practical value in the care of patients and

---

*Now more accurately known as the allied health professional.

their families. Unless the medical student can see a use for the information and the concepts that are presented by the allied professional faculty, he will not have any lasting interest in them. The greatest problem in the incorporation of paramedical and allied professional subject matter into the medical school curriculum is to convince the medical student of the usefulness of this material in his future practice of medicine.

Just as medical school departments of anatomy, biochemistry, microbiology, pharmacology, and physiology have become almost routinely staffed by doctors of philosophy in these specialties, so it can be assumed that departments of preventive medicine, departments of medicine, departments of pediatrics, and even departments of surgery, will add social scientists and paramedical personnel to their faculty. Those who optimistically view this trend as offering them an opportunity to play a future role in medical education should be warned, however, that the basic sciences are utilitarian in nature. The medical student has little difficulty in understanding the application of these basic sciences to the practice of medicine. This is a hurdle which allied professional groups must jump if there is to be the genuine acceptance of the behavioral sciences in medicine comparable to that achieved by the biological sciences.

When the use of paramedical and allied professional personnel in the medical school is considered, serious thought must be given to the degree to which one might be "gilding the lily" merely to keep up with the trends of the times. Unless it can be clearly established that allied professional groups can make a contribution that is unique and essential, there is little excuse for increasing the complexity and cost of medical education through the addition of more faculty. Today the effort is being made to streamline medical education, not to make it even more costly and complex.

Utilization of paramedical and social science personnel in the medical school immediately raises questions of reaction and interaction among faculty, and between faculty and students. There is a growing tendency among paramedical personnel to reject the term "paramedical." They contend that this term does not suitably designate the responsibility that all personnel involved in the care of patients have, directly or indirectly, and that all should be included under one term—*medical*. The term "paramedical" originated with President Truman's Commission on the Health Needs of the Nation. The Commission apparently felt that there are persons who play an important but nevertheless indirect role in the delivery of medical care, and chose to consider them as satellites, so to speak, in the basic business of technical medical care.

One can think of these relationships in terms of organic, chemical reactions. If one thinks of the paramedical person and physician as isomers, then the definition of an isomer must be applicable by analogy to the paramedical person and the physician. Two substances are isomers of each other, if (1) they are different and, if (2) they have the same molecular formula. Structural isomers differ in structure; stero-isomers are identical in structure, but differ in configuration. One can, from this chemical definition of isomers, state that the physician and the paramedical persons are isomeric. They are different, yet they have the same formula for purposes of definition of function. That is, the paramedical person is concerned with the health of the individual in the total sense, and so is the physician. In this regard, they have the same formula. Yet, they are different. They are different because of primary, professional training, background, and experience.

Likewise, in the functioning of paramedical personnel, one can think of the atom with its nucleolus at the center representing the basic, direct technological care of the patient, and the electrons orbiting around the nucleolus as the supportive personnel to the basic business of technical medical care (Fig. 1). There is in organic chemistry the "Heisenberg Uncertainty Principle" which states that the more accurately we know the energy of an object, the less accurately we may know the position of a given object. The analogy here to the allied personnel (electrons) is that ability and opportunity to be extremely active in a given setting does not necessarily define accurately the position of these individuals with respect to objective in the medical curriculum. In other words, almost any discipline can be brought into the major field of education of another discipline, and be extremely active, expending a great deal of energy and thought, but the very accurate description of "doing" by these various professionals does not

basic, direct and
technological
care of patient
NUCLEOLUS
ELECTRONS
supportive personnel
to the basic business
of technical medical care

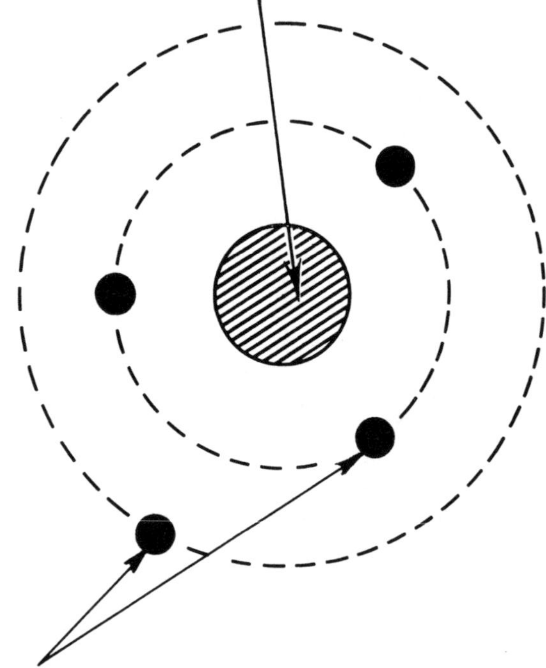

Figure 1

enable us to justify necessarily thereby an acceptably responsible position in association with the nucleolus (the major objective of the educational program).

In the consideration of interrelationships of paramedical and social science personnel, we can draw further upon principles of organic chemistry in the observation of similar professionals functioning together. Similar professionals functioning together would be a combination of social workers and sociologist; public health nurse and medical social worker, nutritionist and health educator. There might be other combinations, depending upon the responsibility envisioned for each one. In general, however, the combinations set forth here are those which usually have difficulty in delineating their respective roles without confusion as to who is responsible for what, and where one's professional responsibility ends and the other's begins.

In organic chemistry, it is known that, if two negative (or two positive) groups are placed at the parapositions of a benzene ring, the two group movements will tend to oppose each other, not unlike two men pulling at opposite ends of a rope, or pushing at opposite ends of a box. Thus, the analogy here is simply that two like professional disciplines have difficulty in implementing the coordination and integration that are so popularly proclaimed as essential ingredients of the team approach that one should expect from such professional disciplines.

Now, if one thinks of the fusion of action of paramedical and medical personnel as chemical reaction, we can think in terms of the nature of any chemical reaction, by which a new bond is produced, this bond being dependent upon the number of electrons contributed by each reagent. This is to say that a new bond would be comparable to a new endeavor and the new endeavor (new bond) produced depends upon the number of electrons (allied professional personnel) supplied by each medical group, that is the medical group being the reagent supplying the electrons or satellite personnel. Here the medical groups can be thought of as specialty groups such as preventive medicine, medicine, pediatrics, and the like. The functions of each reagent must be determined by the number of electrons which it contributes. This is chemically true, and it is functionally true in the administrative organization of comprehensive medical care and research, utilizing paramedical and social science personnel. In other words the functions of each reagent (medical specialty group) will be determined, according to the application of this principle of organic chemistry, by the number of satellite individuals it has. However, the source of the electrons taking part in a given bond provides an important method of describing the reactions by which the bond might have been formed, and classifying the respective reagents involved, but not of defining the nature of the bond itself. The application of this chemical principle simply states that the specialty group in medicine is the determinant of the satellite individuals (electrons) that take part in producing a new program or different product (given bond). Each medical specialty group, being the source of the electrons (allied personnel), provides the basis of describing the actions, interactions and reactions by which the new program is developed, and furthermore classifies the respective reagents involved. This is to say that the medical specialty groups would have varying utilitarian purposes for the paramedical person, and by the very nature of program developed, there would come a classification of the reagents (medical specialty groups) themselves who had contributed the paramedical personnel and their functions to the new program. The important chemical principle here is that the source of the electrons, while providing an important method of describing the reactions by which the bond might have been formed, and of classifying the respective reagents involved, does not define the nature of the bond itself. The application of this chemical principle is to say that there is yet much to be determined as to the specific nature of the bond (or program) that takes place as a result of the availability of electrons (paramedical or social science personnel) supplied and contributed by the various reagents (medical specialty groups) in a new program.

Chemically true is the fact that when a bond is formed between molecules, the attraction predominates only at relatively great distances, whereas repulsion predominates at shorter distances. It is an interesting analogy that can be made between this principle of organic chemistry and the present attempts in medical education to utilize the services of paramedical and social science personnel. It is at a relatively great distance that attraction predominates when one considers the assets, contributions, and unique place of allied professional groups in the medical education process itself. As one attains shorter distances in the development of a program (a bond) these shorter distances oftentimes repel the anticipated potential that existed when attraction was dominant at a relatively great distance. This is simply to say that the application of the principles of organic chemistry tells us that careful scrutiny of the place of the social science and paramedical person in medical education does not leave us entirely enthused about the unique contribution that these individuals may make at the present time. Any deficit, or lack of enthusiasm, as to the potential is not related to the individuals themselves. There is a deficit in the graduate programs for these allied professional persons. Given improved and tailored programs at the graduate level for these potentially allied professional groups, there would be sustained attraction in the formation of a bond (program in teaching), once the individual was suitably prepared for a particular role in medical education and research.

Just as principles of organic chemistry can be applied in illustrating the problems that currently exist in the application of social science and paramedical professions to the medical education process, so can a principle of organic chemistry illustrate the common denominator that exists between paramedical and medical personnel. For example, the formulae below represent three different bromobenzenesulfonic acids. On fusion with sodium hydroxide, one gets the same disodium salt of resorcinol. See Figure 2.

The analogy here is that the sodium salts of the three bromobenzenesulfonic acids are different. Basically, they have the same benzene structure, and they each have a bromide attached. Yet, they are different because of the location in the organic chemistry formula of the sulphonic radical. This different location of the sulfonic radical can be considered to represent a different professional discipline engaged in a common program of medical education or medical care. The paraposition might represent the public health nurse; the orthoposition, the health educator; the metaposition, the social worker, and so forth. Yet, they have a common bond because of their basic structure. The factor which enables them to produce the same reagent is the addition of sodium hydroxide. Sodium hydroxide may be considered to be the physician who is the coordinator, the integrator, and the

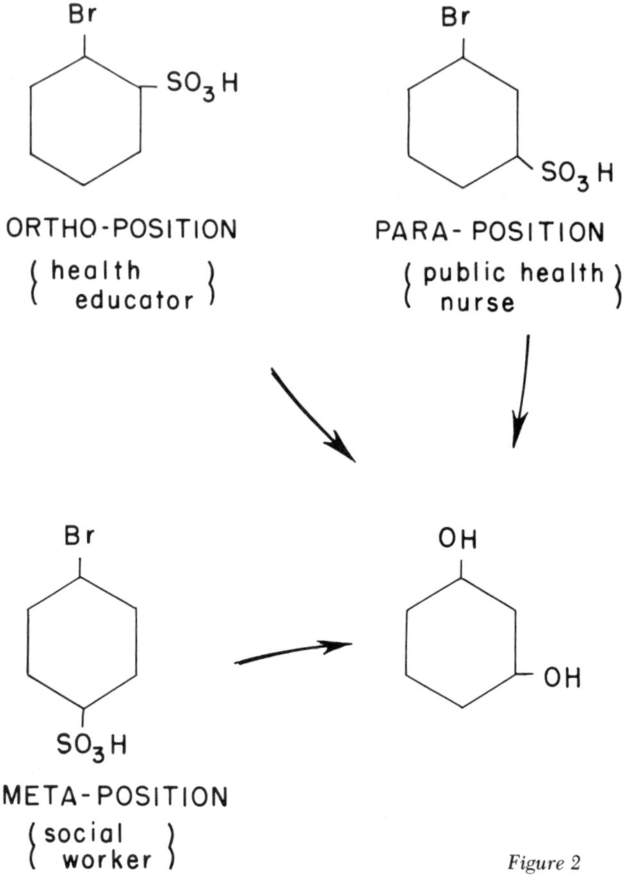

Br

SO_3H

ORTHO-POSITION

(health educator)

Br

SO_3H

PARA-POSITION

(public health nurse)

Br

SO_3H

META-POSITION

(social worker)

OH

OH

catalyst for producing a common end result, namely comprehensive medical care, here represented by the common end product of resorcinol.

In this general discussion of the roles of paramedical and social science personnel, one cannot fail to take note of the importance of interdisciplinary action and reaction. Close observation leads one to the conclusion that there is today a great deal of status-seeking with the opening to a variety of other professional personnel of the doors of a field which has always been highly geared to specific training for teaching and service. The future in medical education of the paramedical and social science person can be determined as much by the role created by the individual professional group as by those who have traditionally decided who shall make contributions to the medical education process. Perhaps the all-too-human tendency to work hard and selfishly for status in a new field of endeavor is less desirable than a critical analysis of the profession's potential for making a meaningful contribution.

Certain characteristics disqualify representatives of any allied group for participation in the medical education process. Among these are disappointments in earlier career achievement. Medical education is not the best field of endeavor for a person who has aspired to become a physician but who has for one reason or another failed.

This leads one to the importance of the meaning of titles, with particular reference to the term "doctor." A desire to be identified with a profession that is held in such general high esteem is understandable. But the greatest service to it will be given by mature persons who are happy with their choice of professional vocation, and who wish to participate in medical education solely for the contribution which their own field can make. Such people will be adamant in maintaining their own professional identities.

In an educational program in which professionals other than physicians are utilized, it must always remain clear that these persons are participating only because they have unique contributions to make. The program is not to provide a platform on which would-be physicians can function with an aura of medical responsibility. This is an important distinction that will enable the medical student to accept the positions of allied professional personnel in the practice of comprehensive medical care, and overcome any antagonism he might feel toward individuals or programs that presuppose an equitable technical relationship. In a medical school, the dominant figure must inevitably be the physician because of the very purpose of the medical school. Allied professional personnel who attempt to function in the medical school setting must accept the fact that many years will have to elapse before the behavioral and social sciences will have acquired the utilitarian meaning that the basic sciences took so long to acquire.

That paramedical and social science personnel can help to produce the kind of physician that tomorrow's world will need is not a matter of doubt. There is, however, serious doubt whether the members of these various disciplines are being adequately prepared for responsible roles in medical education. This doubt does not apply to research activity, particularly that of the social scientist. There is no question about the tremendous contributions the social scientist can make, particularly in research dealing with long-term illness and with social diseases which are no longer confined to venereal diseases. The social diseases of today include those that are related to the cardiovascular and nervous systems, and reflect the economic and cultural pressures of a technological age in a densely populated and unsettled world.

The primary function of a medical school is teaching physicians how to teach. There follows, therefore, the impotant element of health education.

Health education as a professional discipline is by no means new. As early as 1919 the Child Health Organization was founded, leading to the establishment of the American Child Health Association in 1922. In 1922 a section on health education with the American Public Health Association was established. In spite of this long history, however, the formal involvement of health education in medical care as such is relatively new. And even more recent is the consideration of health education as such in the medical curriculum. In speaking of health education, it is important to differentiate between health education and health instruction, for the health educator must do much more than merely provide information. The *education* aspect should be the dominant feature of health education efforts. The scientific approach to attitudes, attitude change, and motivation for positive and desirable action on the part of the instructed, becomes the major objective of the health educator. In the accomplishment of this objective, there is interprofessional dependency, just as there is interprofessional dependency in the activation of a program of comprehensive medical care. The health educator is particularly dependent on the social sciences, and can use to advantage the methods and tools of social science. The supportive action of the social worker in delineating the signs and symptoms of social pathology existing in individuals, in groups, and in neighborhoods is a particularly helpful resource for effective health education. Ignorance must be banished if health is to be promoted and disease prevented, but the dissolution of ignorance cannot take place effectively without the basic analyses best provided by social scientists, including social workers, because of the important relationship of health education to human behavior.

In the development of the Department of Preventive Medicine and of the new role of the health educator in a medical school setting, considerable emphasis was placed on the educational aspects of health education. In his approach to medical students, the health educator should appeal to their reason. Thus the health educator was encouraged to stress the meaning of the word "doctor" in his contacts with medical students.

In its first and essential meaning, "doctor" signifies a learned person; one who has special knowledge; one who *teaches*. By title, then, doctors are culturally aligned with many fields in which there are "doctors" possessing the knowledge and the ability to teach their skills to others. This is particularly true in an age of technology in which there are many professions requiring not only the possession of special knowledge but also the ability to transmit that knowledge to others. In the past there were only three recognized professional groups—clergymen, lawyers, and physicians. Today, the term "professional" is used more generally to designate a person who has acquired special skills in a given field. While this use may be justified in view of the ever-increasing demand for skilled persons in a variety of special fields, there may be too loose an application of the term "professional."

Since the term "doctor" means a learned person, and one who teaches, the implication is clearly that a doctor of medicine is learned in that profession to the extent that he is competent to teach others. This means that physicians are doctors because they are learned men having a special field of knowledge and, second, that they are competent to teach others. The term physician, as contrasted with the term doctor, means one who is licensed to treat the sick and who is legally qualified to write prescriptions. To be sure, in American usage the term doctor usually means physician. The word "doctor" brings immediately to the mind of the average American an image of the physician and all of the responsibilities, obligations, and privileges associated with "doctor of medicine."

In this country, a physician spends much of his time teaching because it is he who assumes the responsibility for teaching patients to follow specific instructions. We might then ask: Is this important, since the physician can only instruct, not teach? Some degree of success, of course, will be attained by the physician who merely instructs his patients, but not the degree that can be achieved by the physician who teaches. To teach is to foster and to encourage attitudes that will make the patient want to accept the prescribed course of action. To teach is to educate, and education of the patient is not successful unless it arouses motivation to act.

If we accept the prominent role of teaching in the practice of medicine, we must become cognizant of factors affecting both the acceptance and rejection of the physician's teaching. If we also accept the essential definition of "doctor," we must require that the physician be all his title implies. University-educated, he is supposed to be a learned man, fully equipped to understand people and communities. He is supposed to be prepared to weigh objectively all the factors in any problem with which he may be confronted. The physician—the doctor of medicine—should, therefore, understand the social, cultural, and economic factors involved in the natural history of disease. And, since disease does not exist independently of emotional, cultural, and economic factors affecting the patient and the family, the physician—the doctor, the learned man—should consider these factors as he rids the body of disease or prevents disability or death.

In order to accomplish these goals in the practice of medicine, the physician must have some understanding of educational techniques. The physician spends a great deal of time in teaching simply by the nature of the relative position of physician and patient in the social scheme of practicing medicine. The patient needs to understand the reasons for his illness and the methods to be employed to recover from it. He needs to understand how to maintain good health. The physician, functioning as the teacher, provides this understanding. If the physician fails to make this educational effort in his practice, medical care is unsatisfactory and incomplete.

The need for technical language in every trade, profession, and business is readily understood. Unfortunately, the technical language of medicine is not confined to members of the profession. An important function of health education is to bring to the student an awareness of the need to be switched easily from the technical language used with colleagues to articulate but nontechnical terms in dealing with patients and the general public. That there is an almost unconscious use of technical terms meaningful only to those who have studied the basic sciences and clinical medicine is understandable. But the teaching of comprehensive medical care must include stress on the importance of enlightened communication rather than impressive, but meaningless, use of professional language. The health educator in a teaching role in a medical school can do much to impress upon students the importance of voice tone and inflection, and of clarity in speaking and writing. Much of this undoubtedly should have been accomplished during the undergraduate years of the educated man. Unfortunately, however, this is one of the needs most graduate schools do not take into serious account in the development of proficient physicians.

Perhaps more than any other professional discipline that might play a responsible role in medical education, health education can do more to give specific meaning to the vague terminology of the past that was, and still is, used to express some of the intangibles in the practice of medicine. Such old clichés as "the art of medicine," "the doctor-patient relationship," "the bedside manner," and the like, are popularly used to try to describe the "something" about the "good physician" that enhances patient response and contributes immeasurably to the confidence and acceptance that are so important to recovery from illness and maintenance of good health. Utilizing the techniques of the educationist, the health educator can effectively break these high-sounding phrases down into specifics. Discussion of the learning process, as it is known to educators, can vividly elucidate the reasons for and contribute to understanding of the factors that enter into the art of medicine and the desirable doctor-patient relationship. Particularly is this true if the health educator in his di-

rect contact with medical students discusses the mutual objectives
of physician and patient, and the goals and subgoals of each in
attaining a desirable state of health through prescribed courses of
action. The element of timing in the educational process, as it
applies to the physician as the teacher and to the patient as the
student, provides the medical student with a definite basis for his
explanation of the diagnosis and of short-term or long-term
therapy, always keeping in mind the factors of encouragement
and discouragement, in teaching the patient the course to be followed to reach the shared goal of recovery from illness or
maintenance of health. The techniques of education enable the
physician to bring a proper attitude to the physician-patient
relationship—an attitude neither of condemnation nor condescen-
sion to the patient's social status. It is the attitude of the teacher,
whose objective is to persuade the student to adopt a point of
view and a sequence of action that will lead to desirable results.

In the program at the University of Vermont, the health
educator had teaching responsibility in the first and the fourth
year. In the first year, participation in the teaching of human
ecology provided an opportunity for the health educator to present approaches to groups in the population of varying educational
levels. Here, attitudes, motivation, and results as they concern at
once the physician and the patient received emphasis in the
orientation of the physician as an educator. With heavy faculty
participation, and with limited time in the teaching of human
ecology, it was not possible to explore all of the avenues that
would be of interest.

In the second year, there was only a limited opportunity for
the health educator to present concepts of health education as
such to the entire class. Yet this continuity from the first year
through the second year and on into the fourth year does provide
the student with a growing understanding of the usefulness of
educational techniques as they apply to the practice of medicine.

Participation in the fourth year in the comprehensive medical
care teaching program gave the health educator the opportunity
to translate the discussion and theory of previous years into
specific terms through examples in patient care. The opportunity
given the students to meet with the health educator on an individual basis, or in a small group, enabled the health educator not

only to discuss problems in communication with patients and their families, but also to lend material assistance to students in the methods of proper preparation for seminars and case presentations.

If the health educator is to function effectively in a clinical setting, it is imperative that there be contact with the families in their homes and with agencies in the community. It is impossible for the health educator to render effective service to students unless he can visit the families in the teaching program in their homes periodically. The health educator cannot function, as some psychiatrists attempt to do, as a third party by acting as a consultant to an agency without direct contact with the patient.

The research activities of a health educator can be limitless because of the type of research that is likely to take place in a department of preventive medicine. In the development of the program concerned with regional medical needs, the health educator served a valuable function by evaluating the health education activities of agencies. Participation in consultation on regional medical needs was not a role appropriate only to someone with the skills of health education, but one that could be played by any person on the team, including the physician, the social worker and the public health nurse. It is quite possible to define responsibilities that the health educator could assume in the division of labor, in an attempt to understand the contributions that health education might make to a departmental program. These responsibilities, however, were invariably demonstrated to be activities that could also be assumed by other members of the research team, such as the physician, the sociologist, or the public health nurse. In some instances, depending upon the type of problem, the medical social worker would serve more effectively than would other members of the team. It was not necessary to assign to the health educator exclusive responsibility for interpreting questionnaires to interviewers in a field study. Any member of the academic team is quite competent to perform this function.

The health educator is of particular value in intradepartmental efforts to evaluate teaching. Functioning as an observer, or as an observer-recorder of seminars and lectures, the educator can transmit his skills to other members of the staff with a resultant increase in teaching efficiency. Because of his familiarity with the appropriate use of visual aids, the health educator can fulfill an important function in demonstrating the appropriate and effective use of these media to his colleagues.

The collection of data on students for departmental use, and the interpretation of these data to the staff, are probably best done by the health educator. This endeavor, however, as was true of all the department's endeavors, was enhanced by the multidisciplinary approach. While the health educator might assume the primary responsibility for this and other activities, the opinions and concepts of other staff members were always considered. This kind of administrative cognizance of the student to be taught need not be neglected, however, by a department that lacks a health educator.

Faculty discussion of the techniques of professional education carries a very important implication for the health educator. A health educator emphasizing *education as such* is an extremely valuable adjunct to the college of medicine as a whole, if the faculty is intellectually curious about assessing and improving educational method and technique.

It is conceivable that a health educator, attached to a department of preventive medicine, could give valuable assistance to the office of the dean of a medical school in the establishment of student evaluation systems. Of particular importance would be the contribution of the health educator to an admissions committee in the development of more uniform and specific admission criteria than are now in general use.

One of the ideals of Hippocrates, as expressed in his aphorism "On Precepts," was: "When the physician enters the room of the patient, he should be attentive to the manner in which he sits down and the manner in which he comports himself; he should be well dressed, have a calm face, give the patient his entire attention, answer objections calmly and not lose patience, and be calm in the presence of difficulties that arise . . . all the directions by the physician should be made in a friendly, quiet manner." Health education can help the future physician develop understanding of the techniques that would help him to meet these criteria for the ideal physician in his future practice.

While the health educator did not serve as a member of the Department of Preventive Medicine long enough to permit further exploration of his potential role, it is certain that the health educator can be effectively used in medical school teaching, not only in departmental activities at the medical school, but also in teaching activities on both the inpatient and outpatient services of the hospital. In this setting the health educator can again reinforce the principles of education to help both the hospital administration and the clinical staff provide more effective service through increased and efficient communication. There is a great opportunity for the health educator to work with the clinical staff in group sessions with families of patients as well as with groups of patients. With the assistance of the health educator, meaningful educational seminars could be organized for the benefit of patients afflicted with the same disease, or for the families of these patients. The health educator, in collaboration with the physician and other members of the health team, could supervise the presentation of effective film strips, movies, charts, and literature that would effectively aid in the treatment of disease and in the maintenance of health. Hospitals are missing a great opportunity by not exploiting the potential that health education has for both professional and public relations. The health educator, with his special background and techniques, can do much more than the public relations official, who is often thought of only as a fundraiser. The health educator can present the continuing story of the hospital to the public and devise a program of continuing education for the public receiving service from the hospital. This is incidental to the educational opportunity provided medical students and house staff through their participation in the development of a health education program for both inpatients and outpatients.

The health educator is traditionally trained in a school of public health. The backgrounds of health educators are varied, but usually have some elements of education or biology. There is a need for reevaluation and restructuring of their professional training in order to develop the kind of teacher in the allied sciences that could make the most effective contribution to medical education and to medical research.

The conclusion is that health education is needed in a program of comprehensive medical care teaching. But while the health educator can bring particular attributes to medical education, and is especially helpful in education per se in the medical school setting, the cost of maintaining a full-time position in this field is not commensurate with the achievements to be realized. There are ways and means of providing medical students with an appreciation of the philosophy and concepts of health education that do not require the full-time availability of a specialist in this field. Certainly one would want the specialist in this field to be available, but for the cost of medical education and problems of financing. Research programs can be developed, of course, and many of these could be developed by the health educator in his own field of interest. But the stability of a department must be based upon the ready availability of funds to maintain positions absolutely necessary to the teaching program, not upon research funds. When the latter is the case, there is likely to be a sense of obligation to conduct research first, and to teach secondarily. Unless a medical school has ample resources, therefore, the position of a full-time health educator must be of lesser priority than a fixed, budgetary position will allow.

In a university structure, however, it should be possible to arrange for intercollege cooperation. A college of education could cooperate with a college of medicine to provide the services of an educator who would present the principles and concepts of health education. Since the educator might lack an orientation to public health and medical care the person responsible for the activities of a department of preventive medicine could work with him on a part-time basis, to help him relate concepts of education to the practice of medicine. The sustained availability of such a person to meet with students informally, and to strengthen principles of education in the college of medicine will, of course, be lacking.

It is through intercollege cooperation that a rounded professional education can be accomplished without undue increase in the cost of medical education. The university complex should be utilized in such a way as to make functional organization possible between departments and between colleges. The initial basic endeavor, however, should focus on the total education of the student while he is in college, so that the graduate school will not have to waste time remedying the deficiencies of liberal education when he enters professional training in a particular field.

D

Program and Philosophy
of Comprehensive Care

Before the inauguration of the experimental program—or something similar—expenditure for public health teaching in the medical school was about $2,000 per year. The generous support of the Commonwealth Fund was extended to the university on the understanding that a program to be developed would be sustained and maintained by the university. The state legislature became very much interested in the program, particularly because of its emphasis on a consultation program in fulfillment of the statutory requirements set forth under the appropriations act to the medical school each biennium. A continued active interest in the Department of Preventive Medicine has been demonstrated by recent legislatures, both by appropriation and by resolution. While appropriations, of course, do not come directly to the Department of Preventive Medicine, the stimulus to maintain the program in preventive medicine that has been developed has brought support to the medical school as a whole with full appreciation of the need for the school to maintain the program now.

In the initial request to the Commonwealth Fund, the president of the University submitted letters stating the intent of the university to maintain and support the program in preventive medicine that had been outlined and that was then under development. This commitment of support came, not only from the president but also from the trustees of the university, and confirmed the intention of those responsible to do everything within their capability to maintain a program for which the university was obligated to both the Commonwealth Fund and the State of Vermont. The regional aspects of the program can in the future bring support to the medical school above and beyond that which might be available through a scheme comparable to that of the New England Board of Higher Education.

The pattern was to replace outside support gradually by the establishment of a sound budget within the university. The fact that the budget for preventive medicine teaching has gone from about $2,000 a year to over $70,000 a year in university funds is indeed a tribute to this small university located in a small state. There was a determination to remain, insofar as possible, on the growing edge of development in preventive medicine teaching and research.

The status of budget in the department of preventive medicine for the year 1958–1959 was:

Operating Budget

University of Vermont	$ 77,578.
City of Burlington	15,200.
Commonwealth Fund	38,781.
Medical Education for National Defense	10,000.
United States Vocational Rehabilitation Grant	22,024.
Vermont Tuberculosis and Health Association	500.
Total	$164,183.

Aside from the gradual increase of funds allocated to the department budget by the university, funds from outside sources for the period 1956-1960 amounted to $412,449. This included $70,800 received from the City of Burlington for the years 1955–1959, the contractual arrangement by which the department staff provided medical care services to the indigent of Burlington. In addition, the Lamb Foundation made an annual grant to the College of Medicine. While this annual grant had been coming to the medical school for a decade or more, the intents and purposes of this grant have been fully met by the department since its organization. The total of Lamb Foundation grants for the years 1955–1960 was $33,000.

Within the structure of medical school financing then, an active academic department usually met at least 50 percent of its total operating budget through research grants. Research must spring from individual interest, and be included in a program of deliberate, academic thought and action. The University of Vermont contributed more than 50 percent of the total operating budget of the Department of Preventive Medicine. It must be remembered, however, that the department was carrying a service load by supplying consultation to the state and the region. Yet the number of staff members did not exceed the usual complement of a well-organized department of preventive medicine teaching in all four years of medical school and engaged in research as well.

In 1955, when I was invited to appear before the trustees of the university to discuss the probable costs of operation of the department then envisioned, I pointed out that it would certainly require $45,000 to $50,000 per year. At that time the reorganization of the city service and dispensary program into the present Family Care Unit, and transfer of administrative responsibility for it from the Department of Medicine to the Department of Preventive Medicine, was not contemplated. The important thing pointed out to the trustees was that an academic department must have a baseline of financial security in order to attract personnel and merit the award of some of the large funds for research now available.

In Plato's *Phaedrus*, Socrates asks: "Can the nature of the human soul be known intelligently without knowing the nature of the whole body?" Phaedrus wisely replies: "Hippocrates, the Asklepiad, says that nature, even of the body, can only be understood as a whole." In the age of Hippocrates, people paid a great

deal of attention to personality. Hippocrates was always exhorting
his students to develop solid, likeable personalities. He never
permitted pathological conditions to interfere with his intention of
studying all the special circumstances of each case. Hippocrates
practiced medicine with an individual emphasis, thinking more of
the patient than the disease, of the cure than the pathology, of
the prognosis rather than the diagnosis. Even in those earlier
days, an important aphorism of Hippocrates was that the physician cannot be a law unto himself. He must utilize the services of
all who can aid him. At that time those who could aid the physician constituted a much smaller group of professionals than is the
case today, these being then nurses, attendants, and druggists.

Five years before the Johns Hopkins Medical School opened,
Dr. John Shaw Billings encouraged students to go into patients'
homes in order to learn how environmental factors complicate illness. This and the efforts of Osler, which date back to the late
1800s, may well constitute the first attempts to teach social and
environmental medicine in this country. If one thinks of comprehensive medical care only in terms of the magnitude of organic disease encountered in the traditional setting of the general
hospital, it may be difficult to keep the efficacy of comprehensive
medical care teaching in sight amongst the host of important advances in pure biological science. That comprehensive medical
care has a place in the midst of diagnosis and treatment of patients with complicated and challenging organic disease is not
questioned. But to give time and thought to the patient's total
situation can seem relatively unimportant, or less important at
least, than the application of biological science alone. One must
remember, however, that only a relatively small segment of the
population requires so intensive a level of care. For the rest,
comprehensive medical care should not seem almost irrelevant.

Comprehensive medical care demands the application of
Leavell's[12] principles of preventive medicine—promotion of
health; specific protection; early diagnosis and prompt treatment;
prevention of disability, and rehabilitation. It demands the physician's attention to the maintenance of health as well as the resolution of pathology. If all physicians conscientiously applied the
principles of comprehensive medical care, of course there would
be a far greater shortage of physicians than is now thought to ex-

ist. Applying the principles of comprehensive medical care would create an additional economic problem. A physician who practiced comprehensive medical care would of necessity voluntarily limit the number of patients for whom he assumed responsibility, since each patient has a family, or if not a family, then other special circumstances that would require more of the physician's time and interest. A panel of patients receiving truly comprehensive medical care would necessarily be smaller than the present number from whom the physician enjoys an income commensurate with his investment in and legal responsibility for medical care. Only if the physician is convinced of the importance of comprehensive medical care, however, can he approach problems in health maintenance and in long-term illness with the same kind of interest that he approaches the diagnosis and treatment of short-term, acute illness. The forces of demography play an important role in the shaping of the attitudes a physician must have in dealing with a public that is living longer, largely because of advances in medical science. The physician must be aware that today's elder citizen is as likely to fear the consequences of living too long as of not living long enough.

Allocation of a budget to a unit of organization is usually made on the basis of: (1) the degree to which the unit is considered important to the total operation; (2) the scope of activities of the unit; (3) the number of full-time personnel required; and (4) future objectives and plans. Every academic department needs the assurance of sufficient operating funds to meet its objectives. This hard core of support may later be augmented by appropriate funds for research, depending upon interest and opportunity, but it does ensure that the department need not be deflected from its essential purposes by an anxious prosecution of research primarily to raise funds. Budgetary stability makes possible a pace that promotes sound planning, program development, and research. Time for reading and thinking is an essential ingredient of the academic life if justice is to be rendered to education and research.

Generous funds are available from federal sources, and the return of taxes in this form to local areas is appreciated. It is desirable whenever possible that department funds come from a variety of sources both official and voluntary, that some research funds come from the university itself in order to assure a spread of research activity that genuinely reflects faculty interest in research.

Using the above criteria for the allocation of budget to a unit of organization, each institution can arrive at whatever amount is required for the satisfactory operation of a department in terms of its own functions, objectives, and goals. This should be an administrative decision, free of competitive endeavor on the part of individual department heads. Naturally there is competition for funds, but this competition should be based on evaluation of the teaching program rather than on the number of research dollars or the number of papers published in each department. Stated curriculum hours are not in themselves indicative of budget requirements.

The amount of time given to the patient has become increasingly important in the preservation of the traditional doctor-patient relationship. Technology makes it possible for the physician to spend very little time with the patient today, for he has available to him rapid methods of diagnosis and treatment and a myriad of personnel to whom he can delegate certain responsibilities. Emphasis upon comprehensive medical care implies not a deficiency in medical technology but rather a need for the physician to recognize the total environmental factors that enhance or impede the patient's recovery to an optimum state of health. It implies that the physician is responsible for the sustained health of the individual, as well as for treatment of pathology.

Ideally, comprehensive medical care teaching is not confined to any one clinical department of the medical school. In addition to the biological data presented by the various specialties taught in medical school, there should be concurrent orientation of the medical student to environmental factors affecting the maintenance of health and the reestablishment of a harmonious balance between the patient and his environment. Just as there must be continuing application of the basic sciences in the diagnosis and management of organic pathology, there should be continuing application of principles of preventive medicine in the development of diagnostic acumen and therapeutic wisdom. An understanding of the natural history of any disease, and the efficacious resolution of all pathology, demand that all environmental forces be considered. Yet, medical records reviewed at random in any medical center usually reveal that there was much emphasis upon the chief complaint and its management, and very little consistent emphasis on the total evaluation of the patient. There are exceptions to this general statement, of course, just as there are exceptions to every generalization. But the exceptions are so few, and so conspicuous by their very absence, as to sustain the contention that genuine comprehensive medical care teaching is, for the most part, an isolated experience for the medical student in the total medical school curriculum.

Unless preventive medicine is taught in a clinical setting, the medical student will only with difficulty accept the importance of the principles of preventive medicine in his future responsibility for the sound practice of medicine. In order for the physician of the future to understand and to accept the important relationship between preventive medicine and curative medicine, he must see that the principles of preventive medicine are accepted by and practical to all of the clinical faculty. There must be a relationship between preventive medicine and other clinical departments that assures its endorsement by the clinical faculty. Otherwise, there will be an apparent dichotomy of interest between the proponents of preventive medicine and the practice of clinical medicine.

In comprehensive medical care teaching, there must be opportunity to acquaint the future physician with the skills and assets of various professional groups that can help him deliver comprehensive care to his community. The future physician must understand the strengths and the weaknesses, the applicability and nonapplicability, of the social science and paramedical personnel now available. The physician must utilize the services of paramedical personnel with the same discriminating skill with which he now utilizes the services of his professional colleagues. Unless there is collaboration between the physician and the social science and paramedical personnel who can also assist the patient and his family, the objectives of comprehensive medical care cannot be achieved. While the physician remains primarily responsible for the mobilization and organization of patient care, he must also make enlightened use of total community resources. Otherwise he deprives the patient and his family of the complete benefits of modern medical care.

In becoming familiar with the agencies and the professional

groups that can help in the provision of comprehensive care, the medical student need not learn everything there is to know about the skills of the clergyman, the social worker, or the nurse. He need only know enough to appreciate how their efforts can supplement his own to produce effective comprehensive care. His exposure to them should teach him that he can preserve his relationship with the patient while delegating responsibility for some facets of the total therapy to them.

Because the physician is identified with life and death, with freedom from pain and suffering, and with the very basic biological urge for preservation of life, there is no professional group that can take his place in the minds of the public. While a clergyman, for example, may provide spiritual support and comfort, the physician is usually looked upon as the immediate source of help and the only real intermediary between life and death. The physician need never be concerned about his relative standing *vis-à-vis* allied professional groups. This fact affects the way comprehensive medical care should be taught. Many medical students, like many physicians, are covetous of their responsibilities, their rights, and their privileges, and since it is the physician who is held to be legally responsible for the care of the patient, it is reasonable that they should be so. In the teaching of comprehensive medical care in which allied professional personnel participate, therefore, it is important that it be made clear to the medical student that while his educational experience is enriched by direct contact with allied professional personnel, the team approach in teaching in no way diminishes the rights, responsibilities, and privileges which are his, both professionally and legally. At the same time, he must be shown that his practice will be less than adequate if he neglects to use skills that bring to his patients and their families a full measure of total care. He must realize, too, that the practice of comprehensive medical care need not be so time-consuming as to interfere with his application of particular technological skills that he alone has. By understanding the appropriate role of paramedical forces in medical practice, the student will later be able to make use of them in the interests of comprehensive medical care.

That a department of preventive medicine should assume responsibility for specific attention to comprehensive medical care is entirely logical. Preventive medicine, with its traditional concern for environmental factors, includes within its scope of interest many factors that are not biological. Since comprehensive medical care teaching is not likely to receive interdepartmental attention, it is imperative that departments of preventive medicine assume and maintain responsibility for emphasis upon environmental medicine in all of its aspects. Comprehensive medical care cannot be taught through any one clinical department alone. Departments of preventive medicine can stimulate and encourage other departments to teach the preventive aspects of their particular specialties. For example, there is relatively little merit in teaching maternal and child health as isolated subject matter in preventive medicine. Rather, maternal and child health should be taught as preventive medicine in conjunction with the teaching of pediatrics and obstetrics. Each clinical department should stress, wherever possible, the preventive aspects of clinical medicine in the process of teaching diagnosis and treatment of various conditions. Outpatient departments, too, should emphasize the principles of preventive medicine in their dealings with ambulatory patients. Here is an ideal situation in which to utilize paramedical personnel as *teachers* as well as in a service capacity to the various patients coming to clinics. Dr. Ward Darley (1952)[13] stated that in his opinion the concept of continuing comprehensive care of individuals and families from birth to death, whether sick or well, is not getting very far very fast. He cited five reasons for this lag in the teaching, to say nothing of the application, of comprehensive medical care:

1. Semantics: The introduction of new words and new terms and the use of loosely defined terms such as "patient-physician relationship," "the art of medicine," cause lack of understanding, particularly when the words or terms imply change or threats to the status quo.

2. Modern Medical Practice: The present pattern of medical care is a barrier to continuing comprehensive care because of the fragmentation of patient care that has resulted from specialization, habits of practice that limit interest to the episodic care of illness, and efficiency measures that limit the amount of time a physician gives to the individual patient.

3. Medical Education: The departmental organization of clinical teaching in medical schools has bolstered this pattern of fragmentation, episodic care, and efficiency. The clinical experience of students is almost exclusively confined to the short-term care of ill people within the framework of a specialty.

4. The Patients: The demand for continuing comprehensive care may not be made because the public may be getting used to the shortcomings of medical practice, and because technological advances are steadily increasing the effectiveness of medicine in spite of deficiencies in patterns of practice.

5. Knowledge: While laboratory and bedside research have given us much knowledge that can be applied to the evaluation and management of health and the prevention of disease, we have very little knowledge that will permit the deliberate use of the doctor-patient relationship and the art of medicine in the interests of problem evaluation and management.

An important aspect of the organization of the Department of Preventive Medicine at the University of Vermont in 1955 was the reorganization of the then existing "city service and dispensary" program into a teaching unit for comprehensive medical care. For many years the city service and dispensary program had been the medium through which medical care at home was taught. It consisted largely of house calls and visits to the dispensary, which was operated according to clinic practice by specialty. It was, at the same time, a method of providing medical care to the indigent of the city for which a contract was in effect between the city of Burlington and the College of Medicine. Although at one time the ambulatory, home-care service had been under the direction of a full-time physician, in the three years prior to the reorganization residents in medicine had had primary responsibility, on a quarterly rotating basis, for the service, including the teaching of medical students.

In addition to serving as a clinical setting for the teaching of comprehensive medical care, the unit, it was felt, could also be a general practice demonstration facility in connection with the regional consultation program on rural medical needs. Nowhere in the medical school was there a real demonstration of the effectiveness, the potential, and the limitations of the general practitioner. Therefore, it was planned to combine a demonstration of general medical practice with the development of the teaching program in comprehensive medical care. This required abolition of clinics as such in the dispensary, and their replacement by the procedures of general practice in the office care of patients.

To demonstrate comprehensive medical care and the appropriate use of paramedical personnel, a public health nurse, a medical social worker, a nutritionist, a health educator, and an additional physician were added to the full-time faculty. A general office aide, a laboratory x-ray technician, and a secretary-receptionist were also needed. The Commonwealth Fund very kindly provided additional support for the development of the comprehensive medical care and general practice teaching unit.

At the time the city service program was reorganized into a comprehensive medical care teaching unit, it was serving some 4,000 persons. This meant that six to eight students were responsible for the care of approximately 4,000 people. At that time the students had about two weeks of experience in the program, each student making as many as 20 to 30 house calls a day and seeing as many as 15 to 20 patients in the offices of the dispensary, a building located in downtown Burlington.

It became increasingly clear, as the reorganized and renamed Family Care Unit launched its comprehensive medical care and general practice teaching program, that a contractual relationship with a municipality interfered with the effectiveness of the teaching program. The obligation to provide service to a large indigent population precluded the development of interesting research.

It became clear, too, that there needed to be less intensive exposure to a long queue of patients, and greater opportunity for the student to obtain a profile of community medicine.* In order to accomplish this, the program in comprehensive medical care teaching was increased from a two-week experience to a three-month experience in conjunction with assignments to the outpatient department of the two hospitals. At the present time juniors and seniors are assigned in pairs to only two families, thus providing a two-year experience in community medicine. This arrangement necessitated discontinuance of the sale of medical care to a municipality. Simultaneously there was an opportunity to increase

*This is an early, if not the first, use of the term, which emphasized a new aspect of the delivery of medical care.

the range of economic level of families assigned to the students. Practicing physicians in town are sympathetic to, and supportive of, this teaching mechanism.

After the personnel for the comprehensive medical care teaching program had been obtained, several weeks were spent discussing the various roles of the faculty in teaching. One by one, each of the faculty discussed his profession's particular assets for the teaching of comprehensive medical care. The medical social worker, the public health nurse, the health educator, and the nutritionist each gave consideration to their probable functions in the teaching of a comprehensive medical care program. An important condition was that service as such be kept to a minimum, and the greater part of the staff's time be devoted to the medical students for discussion of patient and family problems. There was exchange of ideas as to the correlation and coordination of effort that was expected. The specific roles assumed by these professional personnel in a medical school setting are discussed in a later section.

The importance of allowing new faculty in new positions adequate opportunity to think about responsibilities and to discuss these responsibilities with colleagues cannot be overstressed. As the teaching program of the Family Care Unit developed, there was continuing discussion of the function of this unit, and comparison of the concepts underlying this approach to comprehensive medical care teaching with actual results. With faculty and medical students alike unaccustomed to the use of nonphysicians in direct teaching, and with personnel who were new to the medical school setting, there were, of course, frustrations. In spite of the weeks that had been taken to develop the program on paper as much as possible before implementation was begun, the realization of its objectives had to be a gradual process.

In addition to the faculty discussions, the potential relationship between the program and community agencies was explored. Community agencies were visited once again for further discussion of their participation in the teaching program on more than a simple referral basis. As the program has now developed, instructors and students maintain contact with agency representatives who in turn participate in the teaching conferences.

In implementing the general practice demonstration, it was deemed necessary to adhere to the principle that only general physicians would be used. Plans were made to utilize the services of general physicians as instructors in the Family Care Unit. Until a full-time, general physician became available, one practicing physician devoted half of his time to the direction of the Family Care Unit. In addition eight general physicians in the community participated on a part-time basis as clinical associates in preventive medicine (general practice). It is important to demonstrate the degree to which a competent general physician can provide definitive care for many of the problems which come to his attention, referring only those problems that need elaboration in diagnosis and/or treatment. If the services of various other specialties are used in a comprehensive unit, it is not possible to demonstrate fully the challenges of general medicine, nor to demonstrate the desirability of avoiding fragmentation of services to patients as much as possible. Certainly one can assume that an internist would provide an excellent quality of medical care. But what one wants to demonstrate is the degree to which the general physician can provide medical care to all members of the family, utilizing the services of his colleagues as indicated, without compromising quality of care.

All of the families who participated in the program did so voluntarily, after hearing a description of the program by one of the full-time faculty of the Family Care Unit, and in 1960, there was a waiting list of families who wished to be a part of this teaching program. The families understood the implications of participating in this program, including the facts that professional personnel other than physicians would be visiting them and that the primary function of the program was teaching. They knew that the service rendered incidental to the teaching of comprehensive medical care was supervised by a licensed physician.

During their period in the unit, students had a variety of experiences with their two families that helped them to appreciate more fully the principles of comprehensive medical care, utilizing the assets of the community in general, as well as the assets of medical facilities in particular. (The two-year program had been in effect only one and one-half years, and further experience with it was necessary before any conclusions about its modification could be reached.) During this two-year experience, the medical students were responsible for house calls transmitted to them through the secretary of the Family Care Unit, and for coordinating their activities between hospital, office, and home.

In addition to experience for medical students, the Family Care Unit provided experience for second-year nursing students of the university. Some students of nutrition in home economics also had some experience in it. The participation of these other students had the desirable objective of getting these students in allied professions working together during their educational days and thus hopefully increased their understanding of one another's professional objectives in their years of service later on. The student nurse made only two or three visits to the family, and participated in the seminar discussions. The student in nutrition made visits to the family and also participated in the seminar.

The objectives of the Family Care Unit program: to demonstrate the influence of environmental factors on health in a general practice setting; to encourage a team approach in the solution of health problems; to introduce students to the resources in the community; and to demonstrate through practice the integration of preventive and curative medicine.

The staff of the Family Care Unit consists of: one full-time and nine part-time physicians; a full-time medical social worker; a full-time public health nurse and a licensed practical nurse, and a secretary-receptionist.

Personnel of the various agencies that were or ought to have been concerned with the family participated in the seminars. Opportunity for the participation of a social scientist in direct teaching in the program was to be limited, but as a resource person for community analysis he was invaluable.

The equipment of the Family Care Unit was like that in the office of the general physician, with particular emphasis on assumed remoteness from hospital facilities. In this connection, there was a relationship to the rural medical needs of northern New England and the consultation program of the department. The records were those which the physician might keep in his office; attention was given to adequacy of records in the physician's office, but not to the extent of complicated hospital records. The laboratory facilities were suitable for screening laboratory examinations, but not for the more complicated evaluations that would more properly be done in the hospital with appropriate referral of the patient for diagnostic evaluation. The licensed practical nurse did simple laboratory procedures. This practical nurse and the secretary-receptionist, although not faculty members, were also a teaching resource since medical students learned through them how best to utilize the services of an office nurse or of a general office aide.

The x-ray equipment available was not utilized for contrast studies but only for chest x-ray, x-rays of the extremities, and the like. Although a fluoroscope was attached to the x-ray unit, students were advised that the fluoroscope was not used in the general physician's office both for reasons of professional competency and radiological safety.

Research activity began after the operation of the unit became reasonably well stabilized. Stability does not mean stagnation, of course, but only that a solid foundation has been established. Research activity could develop in connection with the day-to-day teaching of comprehensive medical care.

During the transition period in which medical care was provided for the indigent population under a contractual arrangement with the municipality, fees were charged for services rendered through the Family Care Unit. The fees were minimal, being one dollar for a house call, fifty cents for an office call, and drugs at cost. During this period when, because of service demands, it was impossible to establish a teaching and research program, it was reasonable to expect the families to place some value on medical care and the minimal fee schedule was therefore instituted. When the transition was completed, however, the families were selected for educational purposes only and with the full understanding that the program's primary purpose was education of the medical student, the fee schedule was dropped. The families made adequate compensation for whatever medical service they received through the Family Care Unit by their cooperation and participation in a medical school teaching program.

To help the student understand the importance of preventive medicine teaching, and to exploit every opportunity for demonstrating the fusion of preventive and curative medicine, the Department of Preventive Medicine should have an arrangement with a teaching hospital comparable to those that other clinical services have. Furthermore, the teaching hospital should obviously demonstrate the active utilization of preventive medicine principles and concepts in both its inpatient and outpatient services. For these reasons, efforts were initiated in 1958 to establish a preventive medicine service (of comparable status with other services) in one of the teaching hospitals. In the course of a year, a service of preventive medicine was developed in one of the teaching hospitals (the DeGoesbriand Memorial Hospital). The by-laws of the medical staff were amended to recognize the service of preventive medicine, and the chairman of the Department of Preventive Medicine was accorded the same rights, privileges, and obligations as the chairmen of other clinical departments. Figure 4 is a diagram of the relationship of a department of preventive medicine in a medical school to a service of preventive medicine in a teaching hospital.

The administrative plans called for the division head to be the same person in the medical school and in the hospital. Currently, the head of the rehabilitation division in the medical school also heads the Vermont Rehabilitation Center of the DeGoesbriand Memorial Hospital, which is the rehabilitation unit in the service of preventive medicine. The director of the Family Care Unit was logically the head of the Division of General Medicine in the hospital. There was need for further development of the occupational medicine program before a physician could be designated as the head of this division.

Although the foundation had been established for a service of preventive medicine in the hospital, much remained to be done. The general physicians accepted the idea of forming an organized division of general medicine within the service of preventive medicine. During the staff meetings concerned with this development the reasons for the general practitioners' association with a service of preventive medicine were examined. General physicians no less than specialists prefer to be part of an organized entity, and usually the most broadly effective family physician belongs to a service of preventive medicine which does not confine itself to any particular specialty. A general practice division in the hospital can suitably be placed, for organizational purposes, within a service of preventive medicine. It was anticipated that this general practice division would be strengthened, and that further steps would be taken toward the elevation of general medicine as a specialty. If this were to come about, physicians in general medicine must accept self-determined regu-

Relationship of a Department of Preventive Medicine to a Teaching Hospital

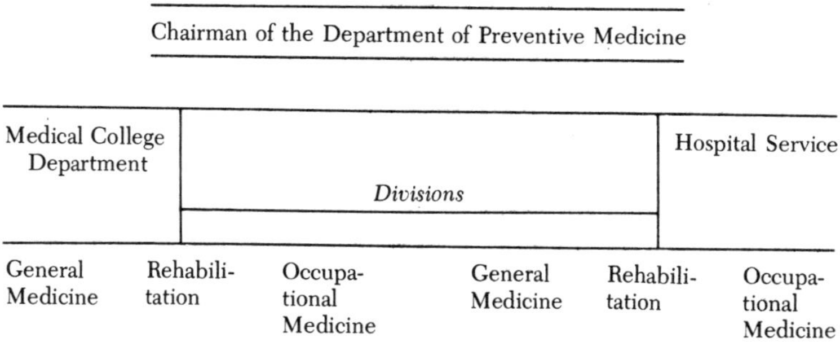

Chairman of the Department of Preventive Medicine		

Medical College Department	Divisions				Hospital Service
General Medicine	Rehabili-tation	Occupa-tional Medicine	General Medicine	Rehabili-tation	Occupa-tional Medicine

1. The same division exists in both medical school and hospital.

2. There are provisions for division heads to be the same person in both medical school and hospital.

3. All faculty and hospital appointments in these divisions are affirmed by the chairman before submission to the dean of the medical school for approval.

4. This arrangement provides excellent opportunity for teaching and research in the department and in the service of preventive medicine.

Figure 3

lations of a high standard. No one classification can be applied to all general practitioners because their training and experience will vary considerably according to their individual interests. A general physician should accept the fact that his privileges in the hospital are granted to him in a variety of professional endeavors according to ability. While he has a personal and private relationship with patients who are admitted for him, he should accept without resentment the responsibility and obligation of the chief of each specialty service to learn what is taking place, both diagnostically and therapeutically, through appropriate record review. This does not mean that the chief of service, or his designee, will actually visit the general physician's private patient but that he will assume responsibility for chart review and discussion with the general physician when he feels, in the interests of sound principles of medical care, that this would be helpful both to the general physician and to the patient. This is the practice at the Hunterdon County Medical Center (Trussell, 1956)[14] in New Jersey.

Much remains to be done before it is certain that a gradual approach to this ideal in medical practice will come about successfully with the active participation of the general physicians. Once a general practice division develops this kind of relationship with other specialty divisions in the hospital, professionally mature and competent general physicians will undoubtedly feel much pride and satisfaction in the accomplishment.

It was understood that general physicians did not receive appointments at the hospital without the approval of the chairman of the department and service of preventive medicine, just as obtains with appointments to other specialty services. The chairman of the service also participated in the selection of residents, and sat with the correlating committee composed of the heads of departments of the teaching hospitals and the medical school. The ultimate aim of the service of preventive medicine was to bring into action at the hospital level, and to extend into the community, the five levels of prevention, namely, health promotion, specific protection, early diagnosis and prompt treatment, prevention of disability, and rehabilitation (Leavell and Clark, 1958).[15] A community hospital that functions also as a major teaching hospital can demonstrate preventive medicine in action, both within the hospital itself and in the community into which its influence extends.

PART

II

The section on the organization and development of a department of preventive medicine is merely an outline of efforts to develop a department of preventive medicine that would:

1. Bring preventive medicine teaching to a respectable level in a college of medicine.

2. Develop this program and this department in such a way as to be commensurate with the functions of this particular medical school, and at the same time, be in step with developments in public health and preventive medicine teaching.

3. Develop a program in preventive medicine that would be functionally integrated into the teaching program at the bedside and in ambulatory care, as well as the preclinical years.

4. Establish a department in such a way as to meet expectations of optimum gain to the student in concepts of total patient care. In this regard, emphasis was placed on continuity of the educational process extending from the liberal arts college through the four years of medical school. Thus, a two-way teaching program as a demonstration between the faculties of the liberal arts college and the college of medicine was established. This was particularly practicable at the University of Vermont because of the physical proximity of the liberal arts college and the College of Medicine on one campus.

There was developed a department of preventive medicine at the University of Vermont which was neither a subdepartment of medicine nor a department of public health. A department of preventive medicine that traditionally emphasizes all environmental forces, yet was so organized as to keep moving with advancing frontiers and changing concepts, had been established.

The careful and intensive approach to the utilization of social science and paramedical personnel gave to this medical school at least a basis on which to determine utilization of allied professional disciplines. The reasons for not including as permanent, full-time staff some of the disciplines which are currently popular in some medical schools are set forth. The assumption was that there will not be the need for long for much time to be spent by social scientists in medical school teaching as such. Collaboration in research and part-time participation in selected areas of teaching are important.

Furthermore, there is something to be said for graduate programs for the development of those professional disciplines that can, and should be, allied with total, medical endeavor. Here, the school of public health is seen as a constant factor, both as a coordinator of programs and as a major contributor to professional development in some fields.

L. R. L.

A

The Wider Role of the University

What is the role of the university? Is it a responsibility which is met only through imparting knowledge to successive generations? Is it an obligation only to develop an ability to think analytically? Does the administration of a university meet its full responsibility to society if it confines its efforts to the university community?

Whatever its other responsibilities, what is the responsibility of the university to its community, its state, its region, and the nation? There are notable examples of individual effort on the part of faculty members of many universities in bringing their academic assets to bear upon problems in the community, the state, and the nation. Should there be, as well, an organized effort on the part of the university as a whole to provide consultation and technical advice on community problems? I use the word "community" here very broadly.

In any community there are likely to be problems screaming for solution that are not being resolved because those responsible are not able to carry out a completely objective analysis. The very human, and often not even conscious, desire to justify the modus operandi of the past undermines the attempt to achieve an objective balance among public pressure, administrative expediency, and a type of commitment and performance that will ensure the maintenance of a comfortable budget.

It is the need for objective analysis that suggests the fitting and proper role of the university in consultation. Since a university represents a body of scholars who are dedicated to objective analysis, whether in the arts or the sciences, every university has within the complexity of its organization the personnel who can, in their scientifically objective manner, throw light on perplexing community problems.

From the local political organization of a small town to the complex organization of an interstate program, there are day-to-day problems in health, economics, welfare, labor and management to which an objective, research-oriented university consultation program can bring untold benefits. Since change is inevitable in every field of endeavor, the change may as well be carefully planned so that it can take place in a fashion that is relevant to the needs and demands of a changing social order. The university, in its detachment from emotional and political struggles, is a prominent resource for the evaluations that can lead to reasonable, long-range planning.

The general public will more easily take the true measure of the university's worth to its community and to the nation at large, if it can see in the university an unbiased and objective resource for help with problems that may be perplexing to the community. It is important that the general public see the university as something more than an institution that grants academic degrees. The university should be, and should be seen to be, an institution that extends a helping hand throughout its community, whatever that community.

In delineating its own "community" to which it will extend consultation in one or more fields, the university must examine its own attributes, including any special areas of concentration that it has in teaching and research. The "community" to be served will naturally vary, depending upon the academic skills and assets of the university faculty, and administrative foresight and decision.

In addition to its own resources, the university must consider a variety of other factors in delineating the boundaries of its service area. Economic factors need not be determining considerations. One is often called upon to help deal with the problems of groups that are under pressure socially and economically because of deprivation, and faculty members of various universities have responded with consultation on housing, labor-management disputes, welfare situations, and the like. But there are also problems in the democratic social order that are peculiar to the haves, not to the have-nots. Certainly organizations with generous resources for the financing of medical care, such as the United Mine Workers of America Welfare and Retirement Fund, have sought the services of consultants, both with and without academic appointments. Transportation systems could well utilize the unprejudiced, unbiased, and objective approach of a university consultation system.

In planning regional consultation services, there is a tendency to think about the importance of centralization, not only functionally but geographically. But if there is an urgent need, and this need has found expression in an appropriate demand, and if there is a resource available that can help solve the problem, it makes little difference whether the functionally centralized consulting agency is also centralized geographically. While it may give rise to some inconvenience in lines of communication, particularly with respect to travel, location of a logical resource for consultation on the periphery of a region does not interfere with its effectiveness. When we say that the world has shrunk, we are usually thinking in global terms, with reference to ease and access of communication between nations. We often do not apply this same "shrinkage" between neighboring communities and states in planning efforts. In our present state of technological development, lines of communication are such as to permit adequate and effective consultation.

The facilities that would be required for regional consultation would depend largely on the problems of the region under consultation. Faculty members in various professional fields who are willing to become a part of the university-directed consultation program are the main support of its continuity. There need not be additional office space, nor an increase in facilities. Additional files and perhaps some additional clerical and secretarial personnel might be required, but the consultation service need not appreciably increase the costs of a university maintaining adequate staff and auxiliary personnel anyway. There are increased costs for travel, telephone, and telegraph, but they are not so large as to weigh heavily against the value of the service that can be rendered. As a matter of fact, once a university has established a sound and effective program of consultation, the related administrative costs are likely to be voluntarily absorbed by the groups and organizations, whether public or private, who sought an unbiased, frank, objective evaluation of problems and appropriate recommendations for solution.

Time and accessibility influence the delineation of the region to be served. While it is true that a consultation service requires time, it is assumed that university faculty members are functioning in a community of scholars where time is advisedly reserved for adequate thinking, reading, and relaxation. Once the consultation program has been organized, the faculty of any department that may be involved can maintain its effectiveness at a decreasing expenditure in time. And, if the objective is as it should be, to strengthen the region so that it can cope with its problems, the greater amount of time will be spent by the people concerned in the local area or in the region than by the university faculty and supportive personnel. Certainly, faculty members who become involved in the delivery of "goods and services" in the day-to-day market will be much more effective in their attempts to project the past into the future for students who will be moving into the arenas of stress and strife in the business, professional, and trade worlds of tomorrow.

While there are no criteria that automatically exclude a region from a university consultation program, relationships with other institutions must be considered. This is probably more important in rural states with few institutions of higher learning than in areas that have many schools. While one university may not be competing with another as to areas of consultation, and while the officials of institutions located in a region that is a logical consulting area for another university could be expected to welcome any consultation service provided the area, one must expect them to evince a natural interest in the activities of another institution in what is their "own backyard." Certainly a university would not extend its consultation efforts into the geographical area of another university without entering into appropriate preliminary discussions, particularly if its own efforts concerned a field of endeavor included in the teaching and research activities of that university. Although there are no restrictions in the selection of a region for consultation arising from the factors of population, geographic location, or distances, there may be some that are related to interinstitutional relationships. Much assistance and support can be obtained when a sister institution located in the region in which consultation is to take place is granted the courtesy of prior discussion of projected action. While the university undertaking the consultation program may feel fully adequate and self-sufficient, there are unexpected and unpredicated ways in which the sister institution in the region, even though not directly involved in the project of consultation, can help promote, in whatever way its personnel and facilities will allow, the solution of problems and the development of desirable plans of action for the future.

The potential role of the university in consultation on many aspects of community and regional endeavor is here discussed in terms of a state university. While there is nothing to preclude the establishment of an organized consultation program as a continuing extramural or extension service by any university, whether public or private, the Morrill Act, signed into law on July 2, 1862, by Abraham Lincoln, perhaps establishes the first precedent for the development of consultation programs by state universities. Justin Smith Morrill, who served in Congress as Representative and Senator from the State of Vermont for more than forty years, was a man who never attended college but played a tremendous part in making higher education available to successive generations in this country. He established, as the main purpose of the Morrill Act, a system of higher education for "those at the bottom of the ladder who want to climb up."

The Morrill Act provided for "the endowment, support, and maintenance of at least one college (in each state) where the leading object shall be, without excluding other scientific and classical studies, and including military tactics . . . to promote the liberal education of the industrial classes in the several pursuits and professions in life." To finance these colleges, the act further provided that each state receive a grant of federal land apportioned on the basis of 30,000 acres for each member of Congress. Hence, the term "land-grant" colleges and universities came into popular parlance in university development. Today, as a result of the Morrill Land-Grant Act, there is at least one land-grant institution in each of the fifty states and in Puerto Rico.

The phrase, "to promote the liberal and practical education of the industrial classes in the several pursuits and professions in life," implies the extension of the university's assets into the mainstream of everyday life and problems. This has been realized primarily in the land-grant colleges' creation of agricultural extension services with county agents and home demonstration workers functioning under the direction of a college of agriculture. While this type of consultation service with aid to individuals and to community groups has long since become a tradition, there has not been a comparable extension of university support on a formally organized basis in other fields.

The University of Iowa took a very active interest in the industrial aspects of farming and agriculture, with particular emphasis on farm safety programs. A number of state institutions, including the Universities of Florida, Kentucky, and Michigan, developed to some extent, or proposed the development, of programs which are in effect consultation services to community groups within a given political boundary in fields other than agriculture and agricultural extension services. Some private colleges and universities as well, such as Harvard, Yale, Johns Hopkins and others, have programs of local, regional, and even international, scope in consultation services related to the health field.

This discussion of regional effort on an administratively organized basis within a university deals with problems of medical needs with particular reference to rural areas. Regional effort on the part of universities can, of course, involve many other fields. But the program that developed from the University of Vermont, College of Medicine, could serve as a blueprint for programs in other fields such as engineering, government, industry, and all of the many and varied fields of educational endeavor of the university. This is not to say that the project at the University of Vermont was totally unique. Neither was the effort to solve medical needs on a regional basis entirely new.

Inequities in the availability of medical care services have long been recognized by many authorities as being one of the unsolved problems affecting the health of the nation as a whole. That there are inequities can be seen in the little hamlet and in the largest metropolis. The ever-widening economic gap between the development of medical skills and their application is obvious. The inequitable distribution of medical personnel and facilities among urban and rural areas is equally obvious. Efforts to preserve the old order in the face of an inevitably changing economic and social picture have hindered progress in the delivery of suitable public health and medical care programs to the entire population.

Repeated efforts have been made in this country to meet medical needs on a regional basis. For the most part, these attempts have not extended beyond the political boundaries of the states. In 1932 the Maryland Eastern Health District developed from a cooperative movement on the part of the Baltimore City Health Department, the Johns Hopkins School of Hygiene and Public Health, and several voluntary agencies. The East Harlem Health Center was established in 1921 by the New York County Chapter of the Red Cross in cooperation with a number of public and voluntary agencies. The Bellevue-Yorkville Health Demonstration led the way to the establishment of the principle of district health administration in New York City. All of these developments were not only within the political boundaries of a state but, also for the most part, within the boundaries of cities, or contiguous cities, and counties.

The story of the Hunterdon Medical Center (Trussell, 1956)[1] involves an exciting approach to rural medical care in which the influence and assets of a metropolitan university medical center extend across county lines to join with a local county effort in the provision of comprehensive community health services. Rosenfeld and Makover (1956)[2] describe the development of organized services on a regional basis, the core of which has been the effort of a hospital organization to upgrade the quality of services rendered and to make possible a more efficient and coordinated use of the region's medical facilities. The region in this instance involves eleven counties in which interhospital activity was developed. There are additional examples of this kind of localized regional effort. The University of Buffalo, the University of Colorado, Emory University, the Universities of Kansas, Michigan, and Minnesota, New York University, the Medical College of Virginia, and Tulane University have, to one extent or another, developed programs which can be characterized as regional, but with varying emphases and geographical boundaries.

The Bingham Associates Fund has extended its operations across state boundaries, notably from Massachusetts to Maine.

The emphasis in the Fund's program has been to supply consultative services to small community hospitals without any formal interstate organization, administratively or politically. The program includes educational activity for physicians, and in this connection involves a university's (Tufts) extending its "community" responsibilities across state boundaries. The Bingham program does not revolve wholly around a single faculty member or members and their interest in consultation. The initiative, however, in the establishment of such a consultation and postgraduate education program for physicians of another state was taken by one member of the faculty when the opportunity arose for the extension of the academic assets of the medical school to a neighboring state with appropriate referral of problems to the parent organization (the consultant).

It is not strictly in this sense that regional organization is discussed here. Regional programs should be organized so as to utilize the full assets of a region, and should be flexible so that as self-sufficiency develops or increases, the regional program can be adjusted accordingly. A continuing consultation service through which a university brings its academic and objective resources to bear on the problems of a region should have helping the region develop a state of independence as its goal. The service should foster self-evaluation and propose solutions that depend on "outside" resources only so long as they are required. The guiding principle should be one of diminishing support as the region attains the personnel and facilities needed for independence of action. Even more important is the principle of developing the underdeveloped, of strengthening the imagination and resourcefulness of existing local individuals and groups. The local group should be stimulated and challenged to apply their own resources, which often exist but may not be readily apparent until an external point of view and assistance in analysis are introduced. A university program of consultative service to a region is not practicable if it merely absorbs a problem which can only be permanently resolved.

By and large, efforts in the regional solution of problems have been applied to urban or semirural areas, as is apparent from the examples cited, and from the many programs in which resources have been pooled in order to gain a common objective for the benefit of a dense population—or a more dense population than is found in the rural setting. Because of the difference in density of population, and because of the relative ease with which communication can be established in simpler structures than are found in urban settings, it is frequently assumed that interstate development can take place more easily among states that are predominantly rural than among urban states. It is further assumed that the complexity of the huge metropolitan university does not lend itself as well to the establishment of an administrative base for a consultative service to an area as does a small rural university. There could be nothing further from the truth than the assumption that size, either of the university or of the area to be served, makes any material difference to the feasibility or efficiency with which the objectives of regionalization can be achieved. The only essential factor in the development of a university-based regional program is that there be clear, unequivocal evidence that the role assumed by the university is an entirely unselfish one assumed by the university only because it feels a major obligation to bring its assets to the medical, economic, engineering, or governmental life of its region.

B

Formation of the
Vermont Consultation Program

Why should the University of Vermont as a state university assume any responsibility for activity in consultation beyond its state borders? Why should a medical school become directly concerned for the medical needs of communities at all? What is there in the development of a department of preventive medicine that would logically include consultation services, not only locally for its own stimulus, but throughout the state and across state borders into two neighboring states?

The statutes of Vermont set forth in clear and unmistakable language the responsibility of the University of Vermont in meeting its obligation to the people of the state through its medical school. Act No. 210, Section 2, as enacted by the General Assembly of the State of Vermont in 1953, reiterates this obligation and states in part: Moneys appropriated for the use of the college of medicine "shall be used to furnish clinical facilities. . . ; to cooperate with rural communities in procuring the services of physicians and other medical needs; and for . . . the prosecution of research into the cause, prevention and control of disease."

Clearly, then, the University of Vermont, College of Medicine, was expected to serve its region and not merely its students. A number of considerations suggested its broader role:

1. A state university has specific responsibilities to a political unit—service beyond the education of its people.

2. Through the interest and efforts of the President of the University of Vermont,* the New England Higher Education Compact was becoming a reality.

3. The State of New Hampshire was already participating in the New England Higher Education Compact, sending four students to the University of Vermont's medical school under the provisions of that compact.

These thoughts, relating to the entire university, provided a framework in which the role of a new department of preventive medicine could be defined. What kind of a department was this one to be? Surely it should be organized in such a way as to assure total patient care teaching, with its strength of action based on a *system* of organization and function rather than on specific faculty members. Its program should be balanced among public health, environmental medicine, and medical care problems. Its function should be consonant with the activity of a state university—teaching, research, and service. In scope, its activity should be related to northern New England.

At this point, the task was thrown against a wide screen, with the consultation function developing as a major part of the development of the entire department to satisfy the obligation of service incumbent upon the university. Since a medical school should not become involved in the corporate practice of medicine (and it is interesting to note that in the development of the consultation program the question of corporate practice of medicine by the medical school was raised), its service function should parallel the extension services so well run by colleges of agriculture. Service, then, was to consist of consultation, based on need for research in the field in order to better perform the principal and primary function of teaching. The college of medicine must relate to a health department to avoid duplicating services and exercising prerogatives not properly its own, at the same time

*Then Carl W. Borgmann.

meeting its responsibility as an integral part of a state university. Similarly, it must be well aware of the role of practicing physicians in the region, respecting their rights and privileges and avoiding cross-purpose action. As long as the service element remains on research toward better teaching, a college of medicine in a state university, or in a private university, will fulfill its proper role with the support of all groups concerned. Whatever the prerogatives and responsibilities of a state university, it best benefits the communities of a region when it responds to invitation rather than imposes its services, however useful and effective the university may deem them to be.

With the philosophy established, the next step was to develop a plan of approach. Certainly there would be valleys of temporary arrest and reversal ahead. Nevertheless, the relationship of a college of medicine within a state university to its own state and to neighboring states lacking such a facility, if carefully and logically developed, would result in steady movement toward objectives. The only time factor affecting the development was the need to fulfill an obligation toward those who had placed a trust in the possibility that such a regional consultation program could be implemented. The Commonwealth Fund had done so, and provided adequate financing for the development of a department of preventive medicine which would both establish teaching and research services within the medical school itself, and inaugurate the regional program. Its support assured us of four years in which to demonstrate whether this could be successfully done. The preliminary thought and travel to make important contacts in the region, and to explore the kind of department of preventive medicine the University of Vermont should have, took approximately eight months.

Northern New England's needs for increased availability of day-to-day medical care in its rural areas was a factor of major significance in the establishment of the consultation service (Fig. 4). It was assumed that a department of preventive medicine staffed with a nucleus of disciplines in the preventive field should be prepared to explore and understand rural medical needs, while at the same time establishing an approach to total patient care teaching that would enable the student to accept rural practice without compromise of professional standards.

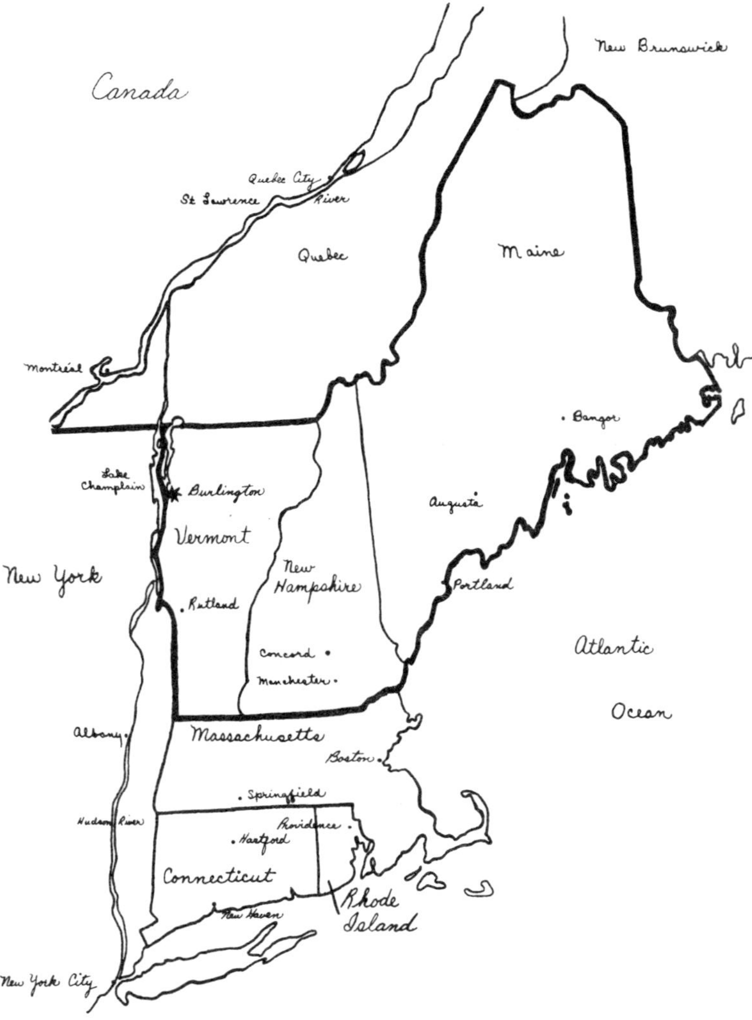

The Region

Figure 4

It was further assumed that the department could help resolve the problem of adequate day-to-day medical care in rural areas by:

1. Making available suitable personnel to study rural medical needs in the region when invited to do so.

2. Furnishing recommendations for action by communities that would lead to the establishment of a physician-community relationship in meeting the needs of modern preventive and curative medicine without compromise of community objectives and, hopefully, in a context that would not be condemned as "socialized medicine."

3. Teaching at the medical school level in such a way as to challenge more graduates to enter the practice of general medicine. The teaching would necessarily be designed to be of value to the student regardless of the field in which he eventually chose to practice. The student would have the opportunity to compare, on an equitable basis, the essence of general medical practice with the specialty orientation.

A variety of personnel were brought into the department on a full-time basis to assist in the development of the teaching and consultation program and also to provide, concurrently, the opportunity for assessing the value of such personnel both in consultation and teaching. The personnel obtained were a sociologist, a medical social worker, a public health nurse, a health educator, a statistician and a nutritionist. There were also one full-time physician and additional physicians functioning on a part-time basis in the teaching program within the medical school. Later three full-time physicians were needed.

Rural areas with problems in the availability of day-to-day medical care were pinpointed as desirable "field laboratories" in which needs in medical education could, both from the standpoint of teaching in the department of preventive medicine, and possibly, the medical school as a whole, be fulfilled. Hopefully, graduates of the university would again begin to enter the general practice of medicine in increasing numbers in the rural areas of New England. Medical education with this as one of its goals must understand the needs of the physician who will practice in such areas as well as the needs of the areas.

Such a broad approach necessitated serious consideration of the roles of others in the health field. The next step, then, which took the greater part of six months, was to bring this projected philosophy of the role of the university to agencies that would logically be concerned with the development of the program. These agencies, notably the state health departments and the medical societies of the three states, could already be considered to have, either by law or by voluntary assumption, the prerogatives of exclusive responsibility for matters of health. They should understand the relationship between a consultation program and an educational program that, traditionally, takes place wholly within the framework of the medical school itself, without involvement in either community or regional affairs.

Visits were made to the presidents of three state medical societies, and to the commissioners of health in each state. These conferences covered the following agenda:

1. Explanation of the philosophy leading to the proposed organization and function of a department of preventive medicine.

2. Discussion of proposed activity in conjunction with the organization of a department of preventive medicine.

3. In the case of the medical society, a request for an opportunity to discuss the proposal with its executive council.

4. Direct request for the president's or commissioner's evaluation of the proposal.

5. Request for endorsement of the program.

6. In the case of the health departments, request for consideration of support in teaching and in the field.

The three presidents of the medical societies endorsed the program, and arranged for a meeting with the executive councils of medical societies. This led to a resolution being passed by each council to the effect that the medical society went on record in support of the College of Medicine of the University of Vermont in its exploration of rural medical needs. It was agreed that plans of action would not be implemented without seeking the opinion of the medical society concerned.

The commissioners of health of Maine, New Hampshire, and Vermont also endorsed the program.

It has been pointed out that a university launching a consultation program must take cognizance of other institutions in the region which have the facilities and personnel for comparable endeavors. For this reason, and because of the strategic location of the Mary Hitchcock Hospital and Clinic in the Connecticut Valley midway between Vermont and New Hampshire, visits were made to Hanover, New Hampshire. The dean of the Dartmouth Medical School, the director of the Mary Hitchcock Clinic and the administrator of the hospital concurred in the proposed role of the new department of preventive medicine. Assurances were given that they would be kept informed of developments. They indicated a desire to participate whenever developments in the area served by them should be presented.

To bring these separate endorsements together into a united force of approval on a tri-state basis, a two-day meeting was held in May 1955 at the University of Vermont for discussion of the proposed program.

At the end of this two-day meeting, a Regional Medical Needs Committee was established which endorsed as a body the principle that a department of preventive medicine had a legitimate and logical role to play in extending its activities and responsibilities through consultation on regional medical needs. (The term "medical care" was used originally, but replaced by the term "medical needs" at the request of the committee.) Agreement had been reached that a department of preventive medicine must extend itself into the environment, if it is effectively to understand and to teach environmental medicine. While the development of traditional laboratory-type of research was expected, particularly in conjunction with other clinical departments, it was agreed that the staff of a department of preventive medicine must also deal with environmental problems in the "raw state" to realize their full potential for teaching. In so doing, the staff might also do much to foster greater availability of medical care in a comprehensive sense without usurping the prerogatives of those holding the primary responsibility for the availability and adequacy of medical services.

The Regional Medical Needs Committee came into being after nine months and some 12,000 miles of travel by auto through northern New England. It was set up to serve as a continuing advisory group to the Department of Preventive Medicine in its efforts to establish a consultation program for the Northeast.

Because the regional medical needs program was based on the premise that the activity of the staff in the region would be of the first importance to the college's teaching and research programs, the chairman of the medical school curriculum committee participated in the two-day session and continued to serve as a member of the permanent committee on regional medical needs.

Because of the tremendous effort and seriousness of purpose with which these men discussed an important development for the University of Vermont, it is fitting that they should be identified as the first organized, interstate, advisory committee to a medical school in the development of a university program. This is particularly appropriate because of a later development—the establishment of the Regional Medical Needs Board as a quasi-official agency of northern New England. The men present at the first meeting in which the Committee on Regional Medical Needs was formally established were:

Robert B. Aiken, M.D.,
former Commissioner of Health
State of Vermont, Burlington, Vermont

Howard J. Farmer,* M.D.,
President
Vermont Medical Society, St. Johnsbury, Vermont

Dean Fisher, M.D.,
Commissioner
Maine Department of Health and Welfare, Augusta, Maine

Leroy Ford, M.D.,
Vice President
New Hampshire Medical Society, Keene, New Hampshire

Daniel F. Hanley, M.D.,
Executive Director
Maine Medical Association, Brunswick, Maine

W. Douglas Lindsay,* M.D.,
President-Elect
Vermont Medical Society, Montpelier, Vermont

William E. Mahaney, M.D.,
President
Maine Medical Society, Saco, Maine

*Deceased

Raymond H. Marcotte,
President
New Hampshire Medical Society, Nashua, New Hampshire

George A. Schumacher, M.D.,
former Chairman, Medical Curriculum Committee,
University of Vermont,
College of Medicine, Burlington, Vermont;

Rolf C. Syvertsen,* M.D.,
Dean
Dartmouth Medical School, Hanover, New Hampshire

Louis Theobald, M.D.,
President-Elect
New Hampshire Medical Society, Exeter, New Hampshire

Martyn A. Vickers, M.D.,
President-Elect
Maine Medical Society, Bangor, Maine

John Wheeler, M.D.,
former Commissioner of Health
State of New Hampshire, Concord, New Hampshire

Philip Wheeler, M.D.,
former President
Vermont Medical Society, Brattleboro, Vermont

The attitudes and activities of this organization were fundamental to any success hoped for in the extension of medical school interest beyond university walls. The events of those two days in May 1955 and subsequent events prompted by the conscientiousness and seriousness of purpose of these officials and representatives of the guardians of the health of the people, made the role of the Regional Medical Needs Committee one of great value and assistance in developing regional activity to meet medical needs.

At its first meeting, the Regional Medical Needs Committee agreed upon the following conclusions:

1. In the medical school's effort to assist in providing better medical services to the three states, it was agreed that:

*Deceased

a. The medical school's primary function is teaching and research.

b. Continued contacts with the commissioners of health in order to provide better medical care are desirable.

c. Contacts with organized medicine be retained in order to provide better medical care.

2. The teaching program for medical students should be extended into health departments, hospitals, and communities of all three states. This would benefit the practicing physician as well as the medical student.

3. Resource material and personnel are available in health departments and state medical societies to assist in the evaluation of personnel needs and the identification of problem areas in medical care.

4. Federal funds should be used for exploration only, not for the implementation of specific programs. (This was a reflection of concern that the new organization at the University of Vermont might be leading toward the development of either "socialized medicine," or the corporate practice of medicine by the medical school.) Subsequent support and effort on the part of the three medical societies testify to the removal of this concern. It was a concern which was readily understood in light of the position of the American Medical Association concerning the preservation of capitalistic individualism in the practice of medicine.

5. Establishment of a permanent committee to be called the Committee on Regional Medical Needs, consisting of those present, as noted, at this first two-day meeting.

The avalanche of requests, particularly from communities seeking assistance in securing increased day-to-day medical care, testified to the acceptance of the consultation program by the general public, with the full endorsement and cooperation of the Regional Medical Needs Committee. It remained a practice to work closely with the medical society of each state concerned, and with the state department of health, when indicated. It was the opinion of the state commissioners of health that efforts having to do with local requests for physicians and availability of day-to-day medical care, should be correlated with the medical societies, and that there was no need to maintain continuing communication with the state departments of health in these matters. From every point of view, a "team from a medical school" was acceptable to the area. The Regional Medical Needs program proceeded very well according to initial purpose. The desired purpose in most instances had been to promote availability of medical care to rural areas, and there were many activities of this nature. (See Figure 5.)

In the initial phases of development of program, it would have been strategically unwise to have attempted an expansive research program that would have defined problems as a whole, either on a state or regional basis. But after excellent working relationships had been developed with the medical societies and the state health departments of Maine, New Hampshire, and Vermont, it was possible to think in terms of a fact-finding program for the region as a whole.

It is extremely important that the distinction between basic and applied research be maintained in this program. Both types of research are of interest to any medical school department. But research that deals with problems of medical needs at the local level (better designated as "survey") must be conducted in a practical way so that action follows, and not merely for the satisfaction of finding out some interesting things. The program is necessarily action-oriented in this regard, and must remain so. However, there is much interest in the Department of Preventive Medicine in conducting more basic research dealing with problems in medical education, medical care, and the relationship of preventive medicine concepts to the active practice of medicine, as well as in the development of a suitable research and consultation service in clinical virology.

At the end of the first year, consultation had taken place in ten areas of Vermont, six areas of Maine, and three areas of New Hampshire, chiefly concerning the development of rural health centers equipped so as to make it possible, and challenging, for the general physician emerging from a highly technical training to practice medicine to his satisfaction, and to bring competent medical care to the people of these rural areas.

Referrals by health departments and officials of medical societies indicated their interest in making medical care more

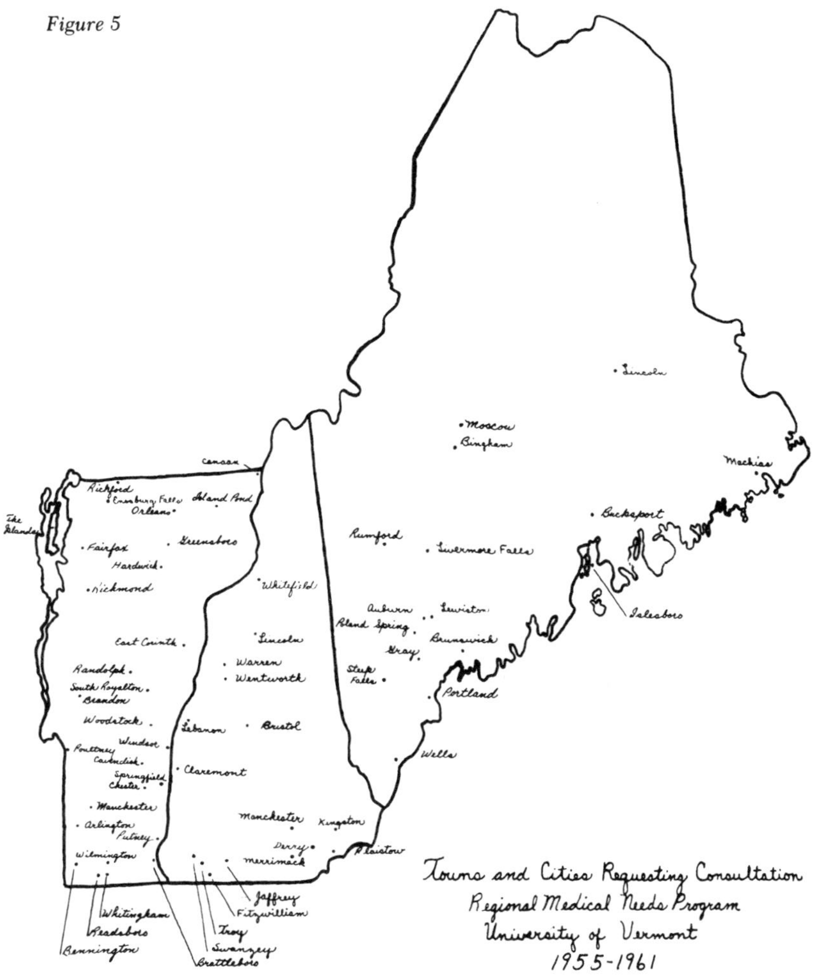

readily available to rural areas, as well as their interest in the possibility of the department's undertaking research in the field. Thus, it was becoming apparent that a university consultation program might well be acceptable to, and of assistance to, health departments and medical societies in efforts to bring improved and more readily available medical care to rural areas. Also apparent was the program's value in the evaluation of existing public health programs with particular reference to chronic disease control. (See Appendix A.)

Demonstrating the services that could be performed, by responding to individual requests one by one, has led to the development of an organized program on a continuing basis. Stability without stagnation has been assured. While the system of working with communities has necessarily had to be altered in the interests of a more effective approach, requests continue for consultation on medical needs that range from problems of physician availability to surveys of tuberculosis control programs, assistance with the development of hospitals, and guidance for the medical service divisions of community chests and the like.

The Regional Medical Needs Board

The Regional Medical Needs Committee led to the establishment of a quasi-official agency known as the Regional Medical Needs Board. Discussion of the development and function of this Regional Medical Needs Board is of interest to all groups that wish to bridge gaps between the functions and responsibilities of official and voluntary agencies either within a state or on an interstate basis. By the time the Regional Medical Needs Committee had been in existence for about two years, the policies and procedures with respect to the field work of the Department of Preventive Medicine had been well established. Medical societies had seen that projects involving physician placement in communities had proceded without any usurpation of the rights and privileges of organized medicine. It had furthermore become clear that the regional consultation program was not a "foot in the door" that might lead to the establishment of either "socialized medicine" as such, or the development of the corporate practice of medicine on the part of a medical school. The health departments noted no infringement on the legal and professional responsibilities of the official public health agencies.

With working relationships thus well established, there was no further need for the Regional Medical Needs Committee to serve as a consulting or advisory group to the medical school. Its original purpose had been served—and served well—for an extension program from a college of medicine had become a reality, was clearly meeting a need of many communities of the tri-state area, and in many instances assisting voluntary and official health agencies as well. To preserve such a tremendous asset for the future development of interstate cooperation in health planning, and such a valuable meeting ground for physicians of organized medicine to discuss points of view and problems with official health agencies, the suggestion was made that the Regional Medical Needs Committee become a legally established permanent Board.

The effort to preserve the usefulness of the Regional Medical Needs Committee on a permanent basis had to be made with full expectations that questions and problems would be raised, some of which might well involve doubts as to motivation behind the proposal that there be any legislation or governmental action pertaining to the activities of a body made up largely of independently practicing physicians. With this in mind, a draft of the proposed intentions and purposes of such a quasi-official group was submitted to the Regional Medical Needs Committee.

In the discussion of the proposal for the establishment of a Regional Medical Needs Board, a question was raised concerning the need for such legislation. Since there were questions not only of the availability of day-to-day medical care in the communities of three different states, but also of the operation of one university in other states and moreover in areas of official public health concern, it seemed desirable and indeed necessary to secure the official sanction of the states involved. It is rather difficult for a group to work in an advisory capacity covering fields of interest that affect the lives of everyone without having at least some sort of recognition. In any case, it was apparent that the group could continue to function as a committee even if legislation designating it as a quasi-official board were not enacted, and that it could still perform valuable functions.

Some professional groups, other than alleopaths, raised a question why the proposed legislation referred only to physicians. Obviously many reputable, ethical, and interested professional groups might well be represented on the membership of such a

board. It was explained to them that it would be impracticable
to have a board so heavy in membership as to render it ineffec-
tive, but that this did not mean that other professional groups
would not be consulted when the occasion arose. Occasions might
certainly arise when a board would wish to consult dentists, social
welfare personnel, employees of voluntary health associations, visiting nurses, and the like.

The purpose of the Regional Medical Needs Board, it was
pointed out, was not to have a "program." It was rather to render
pooled opinion in an advisory capacity on a tri-state basis when
requested to do so. Neither the Committee, nor the Board, was
intended to carry out action programs. The confusion existed because of the extent of activity of the Department of Preventive
Medicine throughout the three states, and the fact that everyone
knew that the Regional Medical Needs Committee existed and
had endorsed this interstate activity. Action programs were, and
still are, executed by the Department of Preventive Medicine,
the Board remaining in an advisory capacity. While the Board itself would not develop programs, it could render advice on programs or on the initiation of legislation that could be of assistance
to other groups in developing programs, or in strengthening existing programs such as those in health departments, welfare departments, and the like.

A question about the composition of the proposed Regional
Medical Needs Board was raised by one of the state medical
societies. The Maine Medical Association does not have a vice
president, whereas the medical societies of New Hampshire and
Vermont each have a vice president. Two of the medical societies
(Vermont and New Hampshire) having three officials, namely a
president, a vice president, and a president-elect, in order to establish equity in representation on the Board, the Maine Medical
Association was granted the prerogative of designating another
physician as a permanent member of the Board. The Maine Medical Association chose to designate the Executive Director* of the
Maine Medical Association as one of its representatives on a permanent basis. Later, to establish equity between the three medical societies, the two executive secretaries of the New Hampshire

*Daniel F. Hanley, M.D.

and the Vermont Medical Societies were designated, by authority of the articles of association, agents of the Regional Medical Needs Board.

The Executive Committees and the House of Delegates of the three medical societies were apprised of the development of interest in the permanent and legal establishment of a Regional Medical Needs Board to continue in the same manner in which the Regional Medical Needs Committee had functioned. It was understood that the Board would have broader scope in that it would be available not only to the medical school at the University of Vermont but also to any organization concerned with health matters or welfare matters pertaining to health. The distinction between the Board's activities and the responsibilities of the Department of Preventive Medicine as assumed under the regional consultation program was clearly drawn. In effect, no program would be started in a state without adequate communication with the appropriate agency, whether the state medical society, the state department of health, or both.

In April 1956 I submitted the following statement of interest in legislation concerned with the establishment and operation of programs for the promotion, preservation, and restoration of health, affecting the states of Maine, New Hampshire, and Vermont, to the membership of the Regional Medical Needs Committee:

1. For the past year the University of Vermont, College of Medicine, has been interested in the problem of availability of day-to-day medical care in rural areas of Maine, New Hampshire, and Vermont.

2. Interest in these areas is based on several considerations:

    a. The University of Vermont, College of Medicine, is the only four-year medical school in the three northern New England states.

    b. A Regional Medical Needs Committee, consisting of the three commissioners of health, the officials of the three state medical societies, the deans of Vermont and Dartmouth Medical Schools, the

chairman of the curriculum committee, and the director of health studies
at the University of Vermont, College
of Medicine (the author), was established as an advisory committee to the
medical school in its regional interests. This committee has endorsed the
medical school's interest in rural medical needs.

3. The Regional Medical Needs Board will study suggested
programs concerned with health affairs that would be considered
for implementation and operation on a tri-state cooperative basis.

4. Any program deemed advisable for implementation and
operation on a tri-state basis would be submitted to each of the
three legislatures with the endorsement of each member of the
Regional Medical Needs Board.

5. Each program submitted to the three legislatures for approval on a tri-state basis will include a statement of administrative and operational costs, division of costs on an equitable basis
for each of three states, administrative controls and methods of
supervision, eligibility for recipients of the program, and objectives to be accomplished in the program.

6. Health affairs are considered to be those functions that fall
within the category of good health as described by the World
Health Organization—"a state of complete physical, mental, and
social well-being."

7. Any programs submitted for legislative approval and appropriation that overlap into the jurisdiction of education or welfare departments will carry the endorsement of the directors of
these state departments, as well as the endorsement of members
of the Regional Medical Needs Board.

8. Previous legislation in conflict with the intent of this act
shall be null and void, as it applies to prevention of effectiveness
in the accomplishment of any tri-state cooperative endeavor in
matters of health.

In meeting with the executive committees of the medical
societies to discuss this development, reference was made to a recent resolution of the American Medical Association which in effect recognized the importance of concerted, organized action on

the part of state and local medical groups. The resolution of the Board of Trustees of the American Medical Association in 1955 read: "Whereas, the medical profession recognizes the tremendous advances which have been made in the improvement of patient care through new scientific knowledge and skill particularly in medicine,

And Whereas, these advantages should be utilized for the improvement of the care of patients,

Therefore be it resolved, that the physicians of the United States accept the responsibility of doing everything possible to improve patient care, cooperate with all groups involved with the improvement of patient care and *accept the responsibility for providing the necessary leadership for establishing joint committees for the improvement of patient care at state and local levels.*"

Certainly, these joint committees could logically be established for an interstate region in which the similarity of problems and the homogeneity of local government, population, and economy would call for coordinated activity, without regard for political barriers, whether county, state, or even national.

Having obtained endorsement to proceed with the necessary drafting of legislation to establish a tri-state compact, the essence of the purpose and function of a Regional Medical Needs Board was submitted to Robert T. Stafford*, then Attorney General of Vermont, who drafted legislation which would meet the purposes of establishing a board. Although Congressional approval must be obtained for building interstate bridges, it was the considered opinion of the attorney general that this was not the kind of interstate bridge that would require Congressional approval.

The draft of the proposed legislation was submitted to each member of the Regional Medical Needs Committee and was acted in turn upon by the executive committees of the medical societies and their houses of delegates. The legislation was then introduced into each state legislature by the respective state medical society. In 1957 the tri-state compact was enacted into legislation, giving official status to the existing Regional Medical Needs Committee as a Board.** The legislation was passed without opposition, the only question being the future financing of the

*Now Senator from Vermont
**See Appendix A.

Board's programs. No appropriation was provided in the legislation, which helped to convince the three legislatures of the purely advisory function of the Board and that the establishment of a broad new "program" for which future appropriations would be required was not involved. Furthermore, the previous activities of the Regional Medical Needs Committee had become sufficiently well known that the legislative sponsors could point out that, even though each state had the "machinery" in its health and social welfare departments and its medical organizations to study and meet rural health problems, the Compact would permit the execution of projects beyond the ability of any one state, and serve to marshal the resources of all three states to meet rural requirements.

Inasmuch as the Regional Medical Needs Committee had been part and parcel of the development of a meaningful and effective regional medical needs consultation program within a new department of preventive medicine, its financing had been provided initially through the grant from the Commonwealth Fund. Since 1959 the Regional Medical Needs Board had not been financed by funds from the grant, and it was now apparent that the $1,500 to $2,000 a year needed for its administrative expenses would come from a dues assessment imposed by the organizations represented on the Regional Medical Needs Board.

The suggestion that the original Regional Medical Needs Committee become a quasi-official board established by legislative compact among the states of Maine, New Hampshire, and Vermont, was based on the premise that a board composed of those primarily responsible for medical care and public health in the tri-state area would be in demand as an advisory group, and would perform fully as valuable a service to the region as a whole as did the original committee by endorsing the consultation program developed by the Department of Preventive Medicine.

While the Regional Medical Needs Board had not yet received numerous requests for assistance, it had had some important problems placed before it. It was still in its infancy, of course, but it is certain that as its existence and purposes become better known, it can become a major influence in the public health, medical, and welfare activities of the interstate region. The composition of the Board provided both a forum at which public health officials, representatives of organized medicine, and medical educators could together discuss problems, and a means of bringing together in continued association these all too often seriously separated activities in public health and medical care. The commissioners of health were likely to have long tenures on the Board. The legislation establishing that the officers of the medical societies shall automatically become members of the Regional Medical Needs Board at the time of election, assured the continuity of their membership. The Executive Director of the Maine Medical Association, as a member of the Board by virtue of his position with the Maine Medical Association, provided an important continuity. The appointment of the executive secretaries of the medical societies of New Hampshire and Vermont as agents of the Board also provided a continuous contact with the functions of the Board, and in their capacities as executive secretaries, this continuity was one which further enhanced the representation of the officers of the medical societies. The deans of the two medical schools change infrequently. The chairman of the curriculum committee of the College of Medicine at the University of Vermont was another member of the Board who was unlikely to change for some time. The practice of distributing the minutes of all meetings of the Board to each member provided all with a continuing account of deliberations of the Board, and the automatic transfer of such records from an outgoing member to an incoming member of the Board constituted a useful instrument of communication.

The following listing of activities presents a profile of the kinds of problems that might be brought to such an organization. A number of these are actions or recommendations of the Regional Medical Needs Committee taken before establishment of the Board, but they would be equally appropriate activities of the Board.

1. The Department of Preventive Medicine had concerned itself with the deficiencies of Public Law 42 (Hill-Burton Law) for the establishment of diagnostic and treatment centers in rural areas, and had worked for an amendment to Public Law 482 to allow an applicant at the community level, as a nonprofit corporation, to receive federal grant-in-aid. The Board endorsed the department's stand that such legislation should call for a contractual agreement between the local facility and a teaching hospital,

"teaching hospital" being defined for this purpose as a hospital that is approved for internship and/or residency training.

2. The professor and chairman of the Department of Pharmacology of the University of Vermont, College of Medicine, was encouraged to establish a tri-state poison control center in coordination with medical societies and hospitals, working with the health departments on the public education aspects of the problem. This recommendation was later amended to suggest that the poison control center be established at the Mary Hitchcock Hospital and Dartmouth Medical School in Hanover, New Hampshire, because the development of a poison control center was well under way there, and the geographic location of Hanover was more central to the entire region. The College of Medicine at the University of Vermont heeded the Board's recommendation, and the Poison Control Center is now operating at the Dartmouth Medical School.

3. The Department of Preventive Medicine was encouraged to study the sociological aspects of rural general medicine on a tri-state basis, including the problem of physician placement. This study is yet to be carried out on an organized, formal basis. Some data had been collected, however, and it was anticipated that such a study would take place.

4. The Board recognized the need for an organized full-time physician placement service in the region with a full-time director. The Department of Preventive Medicine was advised to work out the administrative organization and financing of this service with representatives of the three state medical societies. A formal study of the region was obviously a prerequisite, but it was thought that, within a few years, such a full-time physician service would be established for the region as a whole.

5. The first draft of legislation to establish the Regional Medical Needs Board was reviewed, and beginning with this meeting, definitive steps were taken to establish the Regional Medical Needs Board as a sequel to the then existing Regional Medical Needs Committee.

6. A proposal for the New Hampshire and Vermont Medical Societies to collaborate with the Maine Medical Association in creating a journal, probably to be known as *Northeast Medicine*, received continuing discussion.

7. Early in the meetings of the Regional Medical Needs

Board, the decision was made not to enlarge the representation on the Regional Medical Needs Board to include dentists, nurses, representatives of welfare organizations and the like. It was instead decided to invite members of other fields of professional endeavor to participate when appropriate.

8. The Board took under advisement the problem of reciprocity of medical payment for the indigent among the three states. This is notably a problem in medical care for long-term illnesses. Because of early settlement laws and the independent organization of health and welfare systems and legislation pertaining thereto, an indigent patient is often required to travel a considerable distance to obtain specialized care which is offered nearer his home but across a state line. The Regional Medical Needs Board brought this problem to the attention of the governors of the three states, and requested the cancer societies of the three states to give their attention to an analysis of this problem.

9. The Maine Medical Association for Retarded Children consulted the Board, seeking advice as to ways and means by which practicing physicians could be made more alert to the varying degrees of mental retardation and aware of the facilities available which could be brought to the attention of parents. The Board distributed an abstract of the comments made to the Board by the representatives of the Association to each state medical society office, with enough copies to be distributed to each county medical society, requesting that each county medical society make the discussion of this problem an important feature of one or more of the county medical society meetings.

10. The Board was asked to endorse the international meeting on mental retardation which was held in Portland, Maine, in the summer of 1958. It was also asked to suggest how this international conference could obtain assistance with the financing of transportation of some of the personnel from different countries. The Board enthusiastically endorsed this international conference on mental retardation. Each member of the Board assumed responsibility for submitting suggestions directly to the program chairman after discussing the problem with members of his own organization.

11. The Board gave consideration to the inclusion of New York and Massachusetts. After considerable discussion, it was decided that the Regional Medical Needs Board serves a region

with homogeneous problems of a rural nature which do not consistently or frequently arise in the other New England states of a more urban nature. Further, the Board felt that, if there were a need for participation of any of the other New England states in the discussion of a particular problem, an invitation could be extended to the appropriate organization at that time.

It can be readily seen that hopes and anticipations for the effectiveness of this officially organized group of practicing physicians, health officers and medical educators had not been misplaced. Voluntarily, and oftentimes at great inconvenience, these men traveled to discuss important problems in the distribution of medical care and public health services to over a million people. The Board's experience is inspiring testimony to the potential uses of this technique for the solution of problems and the erasure of the misunderstanding that all too often bars suitable negotiations between professional groups for the betterment of the general health and welfare of the American public.

The Board, furthermore, is of the sort of organization which could be adapted to any region. It would be particularly beneficial to areas which need improved coordination and development in order to realize their full potential in the promotion of health, including the program in medical education and its relationship to the future distribution of broad medical services to a general public. The representation of medical education on a panel such as a Regional Medical Needs Board recognizes the simple truth that the problems of communities must also become the problems of medical educators, if the medical college is to extend its role in the solution of its area's medical care problems beyond the granting of degrees.

The Regional Medical Needs Board, of course, still has a long way to go before its full potentialities will be seen. But a healthful start has been made, and with the continuation of active interest and support, there is no question that the Regional Medical Needs Board could, and should, set a pattern for the regional development of legislation, and the stimulation of programs, that will bring a fuller measure of the values of the technological era to its jurisdiction.

C

Interrelationships
With Other Concerned Groups

The Public Health Agency

Throughout the organization of a consultation program stemming from a university both in its initiation and in its operation, a continuous effort must be made to relate appropriately the activities of the three major institutions concerned with health and medical needs—the health department, the medical society, and the medical school. Formation of the Regional Medical Needs Committee, and now the Board, in no way diminished the responsibility of the Department of Preventive Medicine constantly to show a discreet awareness of the principal responsibilities of each of these organizations.

It behooves the university that sees its responsibility as extending beyond the ivy-covered walls to the community not to develop an "empire" reflecting greater interest in a "big" department or a "big" encompassing institution than in technical and professional service to the community. Since organizations, both governmental and voluntary, hesitate to take indicated steps in the direction of change or improvement of program, there is clearly value in consultation with a qualified group, if financial barriers do not exist. The university need not seriously compete with commercial agencies in the consultation field, but it can certainly bring enlightenment and assistance to organizations perspicacious enough to request an analysis and evaluation of their administrative structure, objectives and methods, and can particularly help groups with limited financial resources. If the consulting university is a state institution, there is every reason for it to render this service without charge to the client, or at minimal cost covering primarily expenses incurred for transportation, secretarial services and supplies. These are the major expenses which would not be absorbed in the departmental budget for teaching and research.

Any college of medicine that attempts to teach comprehensive medical care soundly must necessarily be involved with a variety of agencies in the community. The relationship of the university to the community agency must be thoroughly understood, particularly if the community agency offers a service which is, or should be, closely coordinated with the activities of the state health department. This is certainly true of visiting nurse associations, welfare agencies and the like. While the university must accept responsibility for coordinating the program of teaching or research, it must avoid the dilemma of "being in the middle" in relationships between voluntary and official agencies. The university is necessarily associated with all outside agencies, but is detached so far as the internal affairs of any of the agencies is concerned. Nevertheless, the university has a legitimate interest in the performance of its teaching and research functions as related to cooperating agencies. Its concern with the prosecution of teaching and research can be utilized to good effect in unofficial encouragement and stimulation of interdependence of a desirable quality among agencies. This can lead to a direct request that the university include in its extended consultation program an assessment of the agency. The university then, as a consultant, does become interested in the internal operations of that agency. This has been true in the case of the consultation program at the University of Vermont with respect to both official and voluntary agencies.

On the other hand, there may be agencies which, for one reason or another, prefer not to become identified with the university consultation program or teaching program. The reasons for their stand vary. An agency may wish to demonstrate its independence; another may wish to compete with a university program that has been extended into the community, even if only for the purpose of teaching community medicine. Sometimes this attitude may lead the agency to take the desirable step of becoming formally affiliated with another public or voluntary organization, thus creating greater unity of action between an official and voluntary organization, or between two official organizations, or between two voluntary organizations. For whatever reason affiliation may take place, it is ultimately to the good, because anything that will pull together two or more independently existing groups, whose independence of existence precludes desirable communication, rebounds to the advantage of the entire community.

The state university cannot pursue a program of consultation that extends into the state, and across state boundaries, without becoming involved in the question of appropriation from the state legislature. The fear of competition for funds may become a real factor in the development of satisfactory working relationships between two or more institutions in the state, particularly when these institutions are both concerned with the same field of endeavor. The only deterrent to serious conflict over appropriations in such instances is the early development of understanding as to the particular functions of each of the two organizations. When one of the parties is a state university which is developing a statewide program, it must take the initiative in creating this understanding. Although the legislature of the State of Vermont had shown an active interest in the consultation program which developed in the Department of Preventive Medicine at the state university's college of medicine, there had not been any conflict over appropriations with the State Health Department, the Department of Institutions, or the Department of Welfare, for example. The university's immunity to such conflict probably arises from the statute under which the medical school receives its appropriation. It undoubtedly relates also to the fact that the proposed consultation program did not in any way assume responsibilities of the state's service agencies and thus did not bring about any reductions in their appropriations.

Financial considerations become more complicated when one

considers the relationship of federal agencies to a state health department and to universities. The United States Public Health Service, of course, makes many grants to educational institutions independently of a state health department, although there are some instances in which a university may find it difficult, because of administrative prerogatives, to obtain Public Health Service funds for exploration and development of programs in public health, or in programs to meet medical needs. There seems to be a long-standing relationship between the Bureau of State Services of the United States Public Health Service and state health departments which apparently requires full endorsement by the state health department before the Bureau of State Services can negotiate with another agency of the state. While this kind of federal-state liaison is recognized as usually beneficial, there are instances when a modification of policy that would permit a university to work directly with the Bureau of State Services on a proposal without the necessity of formal clearance through a state health department would be desirable. A university exploring areas of research and demonstration would presumably be astute enough, and have sufficient administrative sophistication, to have discussed the proposed exploration or demonstration project with all the local agencies that might logically be concerned. Appropriate liaison need not involve a discouragingly unwieldy and time-consuming process of selling an idea to every last individual in the long line that extends from Washington to the local community. If a research or demonstration project seems to involve a frank assessment of existing community organization and methods, it is likely to fail to gain local endorsement. Therefore, if total endorsement is a prerequisite, many things which ought to be done will inevitably be omitted. Although governmental agencies carry on excellent service research, and although many fine persons are serving the country through these governmental agencies, a direct channel between the institution and the government agency should be established that could be used for all programs supported by federal monies. The freedom of exploration that is essential to all research and demonstration and that has characterized the participation of federal agencies, such as the National Institutes of Health, should be applicable in all federal-state relationships. This would not in any way detract from federal support to state health departments which have the personnel, time, and imagination to develop research programs within the state health department itself.

This same principle of freedom of contact in relationships applies to the Office of Vocational Rehabilitation. The Office of Vocational Rehabilitation is a federal agency that has accomplished a great deal in promoting the health and welfare of the people of the United States. Yet, dissolution of rigidly maintained lines of contact in relationship to universities would allow even greater strides to be taken in the development of community and interstate rehabilitation programs. Here, the same principle of association should apply as does in the case of rehabilitation teaching grants to medical schools. However, the requirement that demands endorsement of every representative from the national office to the state vocational counselor, is certain to preclude in some instances the development of programs on a research or special-project basis that may well be desirable in improving rehabilitation services to the public.

There are prerogatives, and pressures, associated with human frailties that should not be sanctioned and indeed reinforced by administrative procedure. An agency's administrative procedure should be such as to minimize the human traits of false pride, petty jealousy, immaturity, and egocentricity.

Safeguards have been legislated for programs of federal grant-in-aid, such as the various national advisory councils. The wisdom of establishing an advisory body of expert and objective minds is most laudable. The existence of challenging and rewarding programs in research and demonstration in many fields of scientific endeavor testifies to the ability of these councils, and to the generally sound principle of having a widely dispersed professional group serve as referees in the clamor for federal support of projects in so many fields of endeavor. The various councils, however, are not in a position to evaluate the local pressures, promises, and fears which may influence requests for federal participation in local programs.

Legislative needs are certain to come to the attention of those who fully explore the assets and the deficiencies of legislative enactment. This is particularly true in the public health and medical care field. A department of preventive medicine that has become involved in consultation in regional medical needs must of necessity interest itself in legislation affecting the operation and the future potentialities of the state health department. It is frequently necessary, therefore, to come to a mutual assessment of the need for legislative amendment—sometimes at the state level and sometimes at the federal level. If new legislation or legislative amendments are truly important to the improvement of medical care and public health, then conscientious and earnest efforts to promote enactment are in order. It is, needless to say, desirable to make these efforts with the cooperation of local official agencies. It is helpful to have at least tacit endorsement rather than open opposition, if active cooperation is not forthcoming for one reason or another. In the event of a possible stalemate on a legislative proposal which is considered to be vital to the prosecution of objectives, it is good to have a forum in which such proposals may be discussed. The Regional Medical Needs Board provided such a forum for the regional consultation program of the Department of Preventive Medicine at the University of Vermont.

D

The Heart of the Consultation
Program—Rural Medical Needs*

The major effort in the consultation program in regional medical needs concerned itself with availability of physicians to small rural areas. There were three reasons for this, the first being that the consultation program was established with recognition of the need for increased availability of medical services to rural areas. Secondly, I had, through my own experience in rural general practice, developed a major interest in medical care problems, particularly as these problems affect rural areas. Thirdly, the Department of Preventive Medicine at the University of Vermont, College of Medicine, had a natural interest in the availability of physicians to a region which might logically look to the University of Vermont for its supply of physicians. Emphasis was therefore placed upon the medical needs of communities in terms of physician availability. There were other areas of interest in which consultation services were rendered on request. They had encompassed consultation on tuberculosis control programs, program development in new hospitals, establishment of hospital facilities, activities of the medical divisions of Community Chests or Red Feather Agencies**, evaluation and

*See Appendix B.
**United Funds.

program assessment for voluntary nursing associations, existing hospital procedures, and proposals for programs in gerontology. The availability of physicians, however, remained the major area of emphasis, for it is here that the three states have the greatest need.

The problem in the three northern New England states was not a lack of well-established, well-directed, and expertly staffed hospitals in given areas. The Burlington, Vermont, area, because of the presence of a four-year medical school, has all the specialized services one would expect to find in any large metropolitan medical center. Likewise, the Mary Hitchcock Hospital in Hanover, New Hampshire, which is closely associated with the Dartmouth College of Medicine, has an abundance of specialized facilities and expert staff. Although Maine has no medical school and consequently no formal association between a medical school and a hospital center, the state has complex facilities, outstanding professional and technological personnel, and an appreciable amount of research activity. The Maine Medical Center in Portland, the Central Maine General Hospital in Lewiston, and the Eastern Maine General Hospital in Bangor, all provide a full range of medical services.

In formulating consultation on regional medical needs, the department naturally sought to develop working relationships with these and other institutions. Not to have done so would have been not only shortsighted, but also something of an undiplomatic oversight. All the assets of the region must be considered in the development of a role for any consulting organization. Otherwise one risks the fatuity of bringing coals to Newcastle, or the even more undesirable result that the consultation program serves the needs and demands of the consulting institution rather than those of the alleged advisees. In assisting with local progress in the delivery of services and skills to all of the people, the consulting organization should have as its goal not the jealous preservation of its own role but rather the ultimate self-sufficiency of its region.

While there has been marked progress in the development of medical services in the urban areas of northern New England, the availability of day-to-day medical care in semi-rural and rural areas has become more problematic. Improvement of highways and communication services has not had any material effect. The general situation in rural areas is no better today—and may in fact be worse—than it was in 1948 (Mott and Roemer, 1948).

As is commonly known, the distribution of physicians is far more important to the availability of adequate service than the simple number expressed by ratio to population. While the United States has one doctor for every 500 persons, each member of any group of 500 persons does not have a doctor. This uneven distribution is felt more keenly in rural areas and small communities outside the immediate suburban zones. There are urban centers with one physician per 600 of population, while some towns have one per 2,000 or 3,000 population. In some communities with 5,000 residents, there is no physician at all. These facts were contained in a report of the Massachusetts Medical Society (1960) noting that some 40 communities in that state were appealing for physicians. It is not appreciably better in 1976.

Quoting overall ratios of physicians to population is clearly irrelevant when one is dealing with clusters of towns and villages without resident physicians whose aggregate population may total from 3,000 to 10,000 persons. Replacing a gravel road with a surfaced highway does not reduce the prohibitive cost involved when medical care must be delivered from a nearby urban center, nor does it stimulate the rural population to give a high priority to health needs. A community with 3,000 to 10,000 people must have ready access to daily medical care if the five levels of prevention, health promotion, specific protection, early diagnosis and prompt treatment, prevention of disability, and rehabilitation are to be observed. If economic and geographic barriers to daily medical care are to be conquered, the problem must be seen in relation to the capabilities of the community successfully to deal with it.

In northern New England, a phenomenon which is true of all rural areas in this country—and in other countries—is observed: There could hardly be any doubt that the smaller communities needed physicians' services for day-to-day medical care. Because of the number of requests coming to the medical school from communities seeking physicians, and because of the flow of inquiry from the Vermont State Medical Society to the medical school, it was obvious that not enough physicians were establishing practice in Vermont, without a formal survey and analysis, at least in the smaller communities. Only a study of physicians, by age and date of licensure for practice in Vermont, would explain the trends in physician location. The same deficiency exists in New Hampshire and Maine. The popular concept that the small rural medical school "specializes" in training "general practitioners" for the country is a myth. Graduates of the University of Vermont, College of Medicine, have been turning toward specialization during the last thirty years to the same degree as the graduates from other medical schools. This trend in the country, along with the interruption of service to civilians while physicians are fulfilling their military service, affects the appropriate distribution of physicians in the country at large. There is an even more seriously inadequate distribution, if one thinks in terms of the need for day-to-day medical care to populations along "the highways and byways," as well as in semi-rural and urban settings.

Naturally many small villages that once had a resident family physician as well as a schoolteacher and clergyman, must realize that changes in medical practice resulting from technological advances have made this impossible. Every major advance creates certain attendant problems. Nevertheless, there is no reason why the people of rural areas should not enjoy the advantages of the exciting march of medicine. Rural health problems differ from urban health problems only to the extent that the peculiarities of rural life present varying environmental situations. Life begins and ends in a rural setting just as it begins and ends in urban areas. All of the elements of health promotion and specific protection are needed in rural areas just as they are needed in urban areas. Early diagnosis, prompt treatment, and prevention of disability are as important in rural areas as they are in urban.

It may be that rural populations are a little less sophisticated than urban groups about the importance of diagnostic investigation to a complete and satisfactory solution of health problems. Many small rural areas still cling to the idea that an office call and a few pills are adequate to remove symptoms of imbalance between organism and environment. The noble and praiseworthy efforts of the physicians of yesteryear are in no way minimized by acknowledgment of the fact that theirs was indeed an amazing practice. While many rural physicians keep abreast of technical development, it is only in recent years that physicians electing to practice in rural areas remote from a general hospital have come to grips with the fact that they will need facilities requiring a far larger capital investment than they can generally afford.

Traditionally, many rural communities have offered inducements for physicians to establish practice within their boundaries. These inducements, ranging from a free home to subsidy of income, have become increasingly less effective in attracting physicians to the less densely populated areas of the country. The reasons for this are obvious in the light of rapid and extreme changes in the scientific practice of medicine.

Today's young physician is not interested in just hanging a "shingle" somewhere. He is not likely to establish an office in a remote area where great expense and further personal sacrifice will be required, if he is to have adequate facilities when he can much more easily and economically establish a practice in a community with a general hospital. Realizing this, communities are now seeking ways and means that will give them at least the first line of defense against illness.

In addition to subsidies for the physician who agrees to come into a small community to practice, there are many efforts by organizations such as the Physician and Professional Placement Service in Virginia, the Murphy Plan for Kansas, and the like. Individual physicians themselves have established informal and formal group-practice arrangements in cities with the intention of serving the surrounding population in smaller rural districts.

In communities that have attracted industry, to some extent the industry has provided medical care for employees (and sometimes for their families as well) who commute from the less densely populated rural areas to the factory or office.

Federal assistance to isolated special groups such as the American Indian and the Eskimo has provided frontier delivery of medical care to these otherwise medically isolated groups. For special groups in the population, such as veterans, the federal government provides medical care to those who can commute to veterans' hospitals for specified care, depending upon coincidence of infliction with disease or injury and military service. Not an appreciable amount of the population in rural areas have access to medical care from this source.

In addition to the day-to-day medical care of acute illness, a wide range of medical needs is unmet, if one includes in medical needs the maintenance of health of the population. Public health services, ranging from the ordinary sanitary control of the environment to the availability of the specialized personnel of health departments, are far from adequate in rural regions. Maintenance of health and of a vigorous sense of well-being can be achieved only through adequate, day-to-day, total health care measures which are pathetically and shamefully deficient in the rural areas of a country which is looked upon as an international demonstration of the healthy happy life of a democracy. In Calcutta or Delhi one can easily find adequate medical services while in the villages of India there is much still to be desired. In New York or Boston one will find adequate health services but in the villages and small towns of America there is still much to be desired.

The idea of a health center facility to meet the problem of physician availability to rural areas occurred to me during a period when I was in general practice in rural Vermont. Located in a small farming community of little more than 1,000 individuals, but serving an immediate area of five communities with 3,000 people spread over a 150-square-mile area, I soon found that the quality of service was certain to degenerate because of the remoteness of suitable facilities for even the day-to-day diagnostic work in which a generalist is engaged. Hospitals were 18 miles to the north and 23 miles to the south. Not only were suitable diagnostic facilities disadvantageously located, but many of the people did not readily accept the idea that appropriate diagnostic evaluation was necessary, and were not inclined to travel 18 or 23 miles for such purposes when they were not feeling gravely sick.

The Hospital Survey and Construction Act (Hill-Burton Act) of 1946 had included provision for the construction of small community hospitals containing as few as ten beds, and the Vermont Commission for the Hospital Survey and Construction Act had designated a location about 15 miles from my town of residence as having priority for such a hospital. With the assistance of the late Honorable Stanley C. Wilson (a former governor of Vermont and my patient), Chelsea, Vermont (the site of practice) was designated by the Vermont Commission for the Hospital Survey and Construction Act as a place in which a Hill-Burton hospital should be built. Further investigation, however, indicated that: (1) it was highly unlikely that the local economy would provide the necessary matching funds for this Federal grant-in-aid, (2) if it were possible to meet the economic requirements of the Hill-Burton Act, it was more than likely that the specifications for building and equipment would be such as to preclude economic feasibility for this rural area, and (3) if the small rural hospital were established, it would be difficult to obtain sufficiently well trained personnel to staff the hospital. Furthermore, it was quite clear that the problem was not one of hospital beds, but rather of the availability of diagnostic facilities and personnel who would have the time to conduct the necessary diagnostic procedures. Consequently, the idea of pursuing the establishment of a Hill-Burton hospital in the Chelsea area was abandoned.

Efforts were then made to get the local population of the service area to establish an ambulatory facility that would include space and equipment for a laboratory x-ray technician and an additional physician. But it was clear that the people were not about to "build an office for the doctor," and it was virtually impossible to convince a sufficient number of citizens that they, not the physician, would be the beneficiaries.

Eventually the idea of transferring the principle of the legal nonprofit hospital organization to a rural area for an ambulatory facility began to take shape. I had in the meantime taken a post in another part of the country,* and three other physicians who had started practices in the area had all left after only one or two years. The community, which had enjoyed the services of four physicians and one dentist in the horse-and-buggy days, had begun to feel rather desperate about its lack of medical services. Efforts were renewed to establish a health center, proposals were thoroughly discussed in town meetings, and it became clear that no selfish motivation was behind the idea. Articles of incorporation similar to those of a nonprofit hospital were drafted, funds raised and staff found, and the Chelsea Health Center came into being.

The brief résumé of this development is significant to this discussion because the Chelsea Health Center has become a

*Chief medical officer, Presbyterian Hospital, Philadelphia, Pa.

model for health centers in northern New England. Although it came into being before I accepted the position to organize and develop a department of preventive medicine at the University of Vermont, the Chelsea experience with the provision of rural medical care gave valuable guidance in the development of a consultation program in regional medical needs, designed to assist communities throughout northern New England in meeting comparable problems.*

The health center has been the usual technique suggested to communities seeking assistance in obtaining the services of a physician. For its successful implementation, however, wide community support is essential.

If a physician is needed in a community, of course the people will feel it, and the attitudes of power groupings within the community will generally be in accord with the wishes of the populace overall. Indeed, those with less direct influence in the community may, by the persistence of their demands, bring about the action needed to solve the problem.**

When a request for assistance with a problem of physician availability came to the university consultation service, either through the medical society or directly, the usual procedure was to request a meeting with the person making the request and three or four other interested citizens. The initial meeting provided a sketch of the problem with particular reference to how long the community had been without a physician, the location of the nearest physicians and hospital, an explanation of the conditions which brought about the community's loss of a physician (whether by retirement, by death, or by moving to another community), and the like. Anyone who has practiced medicine in a rural area finds it fairly easy to reach a tentative conclusion whether or not a community can utilize the services of two physicians. Usually it is necessary to point out that the population of the one community is too small to attract the services of a full-time physician, and that steps should be taken to interest neighboring towns in joining the efforts. Sometimes communities have already realized the importance of this because of having

*Phillips, Mabry, and Houston, "Eager Communities and Reluctant Doctors," *N.E.J.M.*, vol. 278, No. 23, June 6, 1968.
**Neighborhood health center concept began here.

learned of the pattern which is followed in assisting communities with obtaining medical care.

The initial meeting with the group of four or five interested citizens led to the establishment of a permanent committee which could be expanded as indicated. If the members of the committee were not representative of the community at large, suggestions were made that additional members be added. Such a committee generally included a schoolteacher, a clergyman, a postmaster, a housewife or two, a laborer or two, either in farming or in industry, etc. While the town officers may be very much interested personally in the project, they are usually not represented on the committee so that there will be no confusion in the minds of the public about this being another project to be financed through increased local taxation. Sometimes, a seasonal resident of the area was a member of the committee, and even if not, one can often be very helpful to the committee in an unofficial capacity. It is extremely important that the committee be under the direction of a permanent local resident and that seasonal residents do not form the major component of the committee, either by strength of personality or by numbers. It is important that the committee be composed as described because traditional role expectations will be of great significance to the community or communities concerned when the hard facts of raising funds needed for the appropriate facilities become the concern of each household. Moreover, the initial committee is likely to be the one out of which is established a nonprofit corporation as the legal mechanism for bringing to the area an ambulatory facility that will attract physicians interested in the general practice of medicine in a rural setting. While a relatively small portion of the population constitutes the leaders in the medical care project, they are the ones who will be primarily instrumental in establishing, and later guiding, the fiscal operation of the health center. Everything that is done must serve to identify the development as the people's project, and not a project of a university, of a health department, or any other organization.*

At the initial meeting of the interested citizens, the story of one rural health center was related in order to give them an idea of the extent to which the community must become involved in

---

*Early concept of consumer involvement.

the solution of its problems. The initial committee is advised that a nonprofit corporation will probably have to be established, if facilities are to be built and equipped that would offer physicians interested in rural practice the sort of advantages they would have without additional personal sacrifice and capital investment were they to establish a practice in a community with a general hospital. If the community has a hospital, the principle of transfer of the legal hospital organization to the community for the establishment of a health center facility is set forth, and it is pointed out that the rural health center need not become involved with the problems of inpatients, personnel, and fiscal complications. Agreement is then reached that there should be a general forum at which the communities interested can hear a discussion of the ways in which rural areas can attract physicians. The initial committee assumes responsibility for increasing its membership and for contacting interested citizens in neighboring communities who should be involved if a project to attract physicians to the area is to be successful.* On a specifically timed basis, because careful timing is essential to sustained interest, the committee is expanded and contacts are made with other communities. Arrangements are made for a general town meeting. Within a couple of weeks the forum is held for discussion of the general problem of availability of medical care, review of the factors which have created problems for rural areas and explanation of the proposal for establishment of a health center facility. After much discussion and questioning the meeting usually votes unanimously to establish a nonprofit corporation, and continue consultation with the Department of Preventive Medicine concerning the establishment of such a facility.

The continued consultation may or may not involve a survey of the area. If a survey seems to be indicated, the presentation to the intertown meeting generally includes a statement that an evaluation of the needs would indicate whether or not the communities could support a health center with two physicians. If a survey is made, this is the first point at which the communities become totally involved through household questionnaires, lead-

*Early concept of regionalization and improved efficiency and cost benefit in delivery of medical care.

ing to further participation when it is time for fund-raising to take place. However, in six years of operation no health centers were established that originated with a household survey.

The survey technique was introduced into the consultation program because of the availability of personnel representing the disciplines of sociology, medical social service, public health nursing, health education, nutrition, and statistics, who had been given appointments in the medical school as full-time members of the Department of Preventive Medicine. The sociologist, the health educator, and the statistician actually conducted the surveys in communities which had requested assistance in obtaining the services of physicians. It is extremely important that the questionnaires be tailored to fit the particular community. While some of the questions would apply in any situation, others would not be appropriate for an island off the coast of Maine, for example. Or, if there is an osteopath or a chiropractor in the community, the questionnaire should elicit information concerning the degree to which these sources are used by the community.

Since the population of the areas is quite small, and there has been relatively little change over a ten-year period, it was possible to do universe sampling in almost all the surveys. The town clerk's office often is a better source of information than census data.

As has been noted earlier, one of the purposes of the department was to explore the contributions that allied health professionals and social science personnel could make as full-time faculty members in a medical school. As a result, they were brought into the consultation program as well as into teaching and research activities, and given freedom to develop whatever approaches they deemed advisable. Therefore, even though the physician in the program could identify problems simply because of his experience in rural medicine and public health practice, it was important that we pursue procedures which, even though very time-consuming and very expensive, might reveal more suitable solutions than might otherwise be found . . . both for rural communities and for the utilization of allied health professionals and social science personnel.

After a number of surveys had been carried out, the statistician was asked to evaluate several of them in an effort to ascertain the size of sample that would give reliable information concerning demographic characteristics, attitudes, and opinions of the populations involved.

In surveying small communities in rural areas, procedures should be adapted to the local situation. In our experience, it is far better to work with the town clerk, the selectmen, and others in the community who know the town well than to use only traditional census data and statistical analyses by region for this purpose.

Because of the tremendous demand for assistance from communities in need of daily medical care, it was not always possible to wait while a formal survey was being made. This was particularly true because a part, and an important part, of the proposal for the establishment of a consultation service from a department of preventive medicine was to determine the degree to which there would be requests for consultation. It was necessary to work extremely hard, week in and week out, in order to discharge our responsibilities to communities requesting assistance while, at the same time, maintaining an active case load to determine the amount of demand such a consultation service might expect. Happily, all communities with which there had been contact have been very much satisfied with results—even those who were told that they did not really need a resident physician. With the tremendous load of consultations, including those from the Burlington, Vermont, area, and the need to simultaneously establish a department to meet the intramural purposes of teaching and research, it was necessary to streamline activities. This was accomplished principally by asking that the representatives of a community seeking assistance come to the medical school for the initial meeting. It was also demonstrated that a committee can be given questionnaires with appropriate printed instructions, and following discussion of these instructions, it will satisfactorily administer it on a self-study basis and return the results to the university for analysis. The questionnaire itself can be greatly simplified and still yield a picture of the possibility or the probability of need, as well as demand, for improved access to daily medical care. This system recognizes the communities' responsibility to work toward the solution of its own problems. It enables the community to recognize more fully that physicians no longer respond to salary subsidy as they did in former years. The community can see more clearly that the establishment of facilities suitable for the modern practice of general medicine is a business venture that will enable the small rural community to compete with urban areas for the services of physicians. Suitable housing, school standards, and opportunities for recreation may be important factors in the physician's choice of a place to live, but any properly equipped rural community that is reasonably progressive will not have difficulty attracting physicians interested in general medicine.

In addition to assisting a community in the establishment of a health center, the university-based consultation service can and did render additional help to the centers themselves. It cooperated in arranging a continuing relationship between hospitals and the health center, in the training of ancillary staff, in advice on the equipment needed in the health center, and in the screening of physicians seeking to rent offices in the health center.

Nevertheless, the continuing relationship of the medical school to the health center was not as active as one would have hoped. While there was continuing availability of consultation from the Department of Preventive Medicine, and while there was continued effort to cooperate in the training of general office aides for the health centers, there had not been much extension of other clinical consultation into the health center itself from the faculty of the medical school. This is an important provision included in the rules and regulations adopted by the trustees of the health centers. The opportunity for physicians of the health centers to participate in the teaching activities of the hospitals provided consultation for the physicians, but it would be a much stronger and increasingly valuable relationship if there were a regular continuing basis for the visits of various members of the faculty to the health centers. Such continuity of consultation at the health center by various faculty members must, of course, have the endorsement and continuing interest of the physicians of the health center. The initial interest of the medical school in extending consultation into a region provides the basis on which the administration of the medical school could approach the physicians of health centers expressly to arrange for faculty members to visit from time to time in accordance with a mutually satisfactory plan as to frequency and program. Such a program of continuing postgraduate education for physicians in conjunction with a formalized program of extension services to health centers could hardly be misinterpreted as "the corporate practice of medicine by a medical school."

Only a family practitioner can solve the problem of the availability of daily medical services in rural areas. Small rural areas are not likely to have a population large and complex enough to constitute a professional challenge or to support the services of a group practice in which specialists are included. It is generally recognized that the competent general physician with adequate professional training can take care of 85 percent of the problems on a definitive basis. This is true only when the physician has suitable professional training, including professional experience beyond the internship, and has at his disposal adequate facilities for diagnosis and treatment. There is no attempt here to define the family practitioner; this has been attempted over and over again. Suffice it to say there is such a person as a family physician, there always has been and there always will be.* Hospital appointments for the generalist have created a great problem, but this problem is probably magnified through the error of including all generalists under one category for administrative purposes in the general hospital. The generalist may be a person who has spent considerable time in medicine, or in surgery, or in any other field—and yet be a person who wishes to be responsible for total family groups, and to whom any member of the family may come either for diagnosis and definitive treatment or for appropriate referral if indicated. Clark (1953), in a discussion of general practice in the future, placed generalists in three categories. The first consists of those who have been inadequately trained by a rotating internship of one year or less; the second, those who have more nearly been adequately trained by two or more years of internship—residency program; and, the third, those he prefers to call "generalists-specialists," a very few of whom have been primarily trained by inadequate residency, but most gradually developed from the first two classifications.

In addition, Clark presents five geographic considerations, namely, urban, suburban, small city, semi-rural, and rural. In the

*Specialty Board certification in family medicine now attests to this.

urban practice, he describes the inadequately trained generalist who works in the midst of teaching hospitals and the best specialists available, but who is not qualified for appointment to the staff. He depends upon volume and low fees, and develops a rapid "spot diagnosis" technique. Under his circumstances he deteriorates rather than improves in professional competence.

The suburban generalist, though sometimes inadequately trained, may receive appointment to the staff of a good small local hospital on a trial basis. Enlightened trustees of such hospitals do not allow him to perform major surgical procedures, but do provide opportunity for recognition through ambition and conscientious endeavor.

The small city generalist is existing under conditions comparable to the suburban generalist. Dissimilarities arise, however, because of increased distance from medical centers and the variation of medical development in the individual city.

In the semi-rural practice, in towns of approximately 3,000 people, plus surrounding towns making an aggregate of 10,000 to 20,000 people, there is similarity to the small city and suburban medical practice, with the major exception being that there are few, if any, local specialists in the semi-rural area. This physician, then, has to be competent in internal medicine, obstetrics, and pediatrics, referring to specialists in the nearby city as indicated.

The rural generalist is generally considered to be in an isolated situation which makes it impossible for him to reach the nearest hospital once or twice a day without jeopardizing his work. Here, too, he has a harder job organizing an office practice successfully because for years it has been customary for rural patients to demand house calls. There was not much point in their coming to the physician's office unless he had to offer there the advantages of technical equipment which would enable him to make at least a satisfactory working diagnosis. Contact with professional colleagues is lacking in rural practice. Consequently, whatever the community does to secure daily medical services must take into consideration the needs of the physician, not only as to his family and social life, but as to his professional advancement and comfort.

Reference has already been made to the Virginia Plan, the Kansas Plan, and other efforts which have been made to meet the problems of the community in need. The methods of solution vary, but the common denominators of professional competence and adequacy of facilities, which include the availability of a general hospital even if it is fifteen or twenty miles away, are matters which are of mutual concern to all of those who work with the problem of the community in need of day-to-day medical care.

A brochure published by the American Medical Association in cooperation with the Sears Roebuck Foundation* is entitled "The Business Side of Medical Practice." It sets forth important problems facing the young physician seeking a community in which to practice. It lists these pertinent questions:

1. Does the community need a physician?
2. Can it support a physician?
3. Can I find a good office location?
4. Are hospital facilities available to me within a reasonable distance?
5. Will I have access to diagnostic and therapeutic facilities?
6. Are there drugstores in the area?
7. Can I supplement my income with other work while building my practice? And equally important, will my family be happy here? Will we "fit in"? Can I find a suitable home? Are there churches, good schools, and stores nearby? Are there social and recreational outlets for us?

The same brochure produces an interesting map showing percent of change in physician population and percent of change in general population state by state. This publication notes that "the development of modern cars and superhighways has speeded up this process so that distance no longer is a factor in obtaining speedy medical care." While it is true that a physician seeking a place to practice is interested in population densities, depending upon his particular interest, it is not true that modern cars and superhighways have removed the need for physicians to be located within areas that have sufficient density of population (2,800 to 3,000) to support at least two physicians, professionally and economically. People in these areas may make a speed-run to the city for an emergency. But, unless there is ready access to physi-

*The Department of Preventive Medicine gave consultation to the Medical Division, Sears Roebuck Foundation.

cians, the foundations of sound medical practice, namely health promotion and prevention, suffer. Consequently such populations go without early medical care—the keystone to maintenance of health.

Once a facility has been established, there is need for follow-through. A group of citizens in a community who have no sophistication in medical matters find themselves in a position in which they must develop an understanding of their relationship to the physicians, to the staff of the health center, and to their peers in the interest of the sound operation of the health center. Physicians generally do not understand very well the relationship of trustees to the hospital in which they have had their clinical clerkships and their graduate education until they have been members of a hospital staff for some time. Similarly, physicians who come to an organized health center usually are not in a position to understand the legal and functional relationships between the trustees of a health center and themselves. Neither do physicians have much idea as to how to go about setting up an office, selecting equipment and drugs, instituting business procedures for accounting purposes, and the like.

The health department has a golden opportunity to extend its influence into rural areas through the medium of a health center that has been established by the efforts of a local group. The health center in the rural area presents an ideal environment for organized public health activity. It takes some time before a group of trustees in a local rural health center are ready to absorb public health programs as such. Once they are over the hurdle of establishing the health center and they see it is operating smoothly, they are ready to listen and to adopt mechanisms that will bring public health programs into the health center. These might be programs in health education and health promotion for the community. The health center can be the focus for improvement of environmental sanitation, and for any program that the health department could envision as being adaptable to the service area of such a health center.

The physicians themselves are usually not fully geared to the possibilities of fusion of preventive and curative medicine, although trends in medical education hopefully will provide future physicians with an increased appreciation and awareness of the gains to be made through such bilateral endeavors.

The community itself has the greatest responsibility in follow-through. Usually there is no problem whatsoever with this, especially if the health center has been initiated as a project of the local area, not of the consulting agency. The follow-through on the part of the community is not unlike that of the follow-through in a community that has a hospital. Voluntary fund-raising efforts on a continuing basis such as are made by ladies' auxiliaries for hospitals can be made for the rural health center as well. Fund-raising is a device through which the community maintains a very active interest in the fiscal and functional welfare of the health center as a community agency. Oftentimes, seasonal residents are very helpful to the climate of the health center through their active interest and support. It is extremely important that the rural health center be on the growing edge of possibilities for community service, just as the forward-looking hospital evolves more and more into a community agency. The health center reaches very intimately into the daily lives of inhabitants in the small rural area. So does the general hospital in its fulfillment of responsibility to a community. Its responsibility does not begin and end with the arrival and discharge of patients.* There are many ways in which the health center can cooperate with the local public health official just as there are many ways in which the hospital can, and has in some instances, cooperated with local or state public health officials. The initiative for such cooperation may come from either the hospital or from the public health official, but in any case it should take place so that the people of a community, whether urban or rural, can realize the full benefits of health promotion and maintenance through the combined efforts of public health and clinical medicine.

This approach to the problems of the community in need cannot be labeled "socialized medicine." The principle of the hospital organization is simply transferred to the rural area. Physicians are engaged on a voluntary basis in a fee-for-service or some other type of practice. They have at their disposal only the facilities available to physicians who have their offices adjacent to the hospital, or within the hospital. It makes unnecessary the operation of undesirable itinerant rural clinics. It establishes a pri-

*Early recognition of the need for departments of community medicine in hospitals.

vate practice of medicine in rural areas, but with an opportunity to combine the clinic approach of a public health agency and organized medicine. It makes the facility something that is more than a clinic in an urban area, which is still too often thought of as for the worthy poor. It is under the sponsorship of a voluntary, nonprofit body.

The true health center for the community in need of daily medical services provides the medium through which the World Health Organization definition of health can be simply applied, giving to each individual as it does a complete state of physical, social, and mental well-being. Only a beginning had been made, but it was an important beginning toward the solution of rural medical care problems. With increased effort, and increased communication and cooperative endeavor among universities, medical societies, and health departments, an administratively feasible mechanism can be established for the delivery of comprehensive medical service. There are other organizations without whose cooperation and interest the distance between reach and grasp cannot be shortened—dental societies, welfare organizations, and proprietors of nursing homes and homes for the aged.

E

Role of Paramedical
Personnel in Consultation Service

The Physician

For a physician to function in field consultation in a program of public health and medical care, he needs to have training and experience beyond his technical understanding of medicine. Too often, the assumption is made by physicians themselves, and by others, that because this individual has met the requirements of licensure for the practice of medicine, he is equipped to deal with problems in public health practice and in problems of delivery of medical care according to local or regional needs. While an understanding of the technology of the practice of medicine is indispensable to sound medical administration and to sound public health practice, technical training in medicine alone is insufficient to understand and to deal with problems in public health and medical care.

Physicians in general are seriously deficient in an understanding of the many media through which medical care is provided. For the physician to function in a department of preventive medicine that has a consultation program, he should have a working knowledge of these many media including the solo physician's office, the hospital, the administrative complexities of nursing homes, convalescent centers, rehabilitation facilities, and the like. There cannot be an adequate understanding of these many media without some knowledge of the impact of political and legislative machinations of our society. The physician involved in a full-time, academic position should have some understanding of legislative machinery, and be familiar with the legal interpretation of public health laws and regulations.

Since preventive medicine is not confined to any one clinical specialty, the physician engaged in the full-time pursuit of preventive medicine activities is better equipped for these responsibilities if he has a broad, general view of medical activity. Emphasis in internal medicine, pediatrics, surgery or obstetrics, or in any other field, does not in itself better prepare the physician as a full-time member of a department of preventive medicine. Basic disciplines of epidemiology and public health practice will serve to give the full-time physician in preventive medicine, regardless of any special interest which he may have, a reference point for fact-finding and solution. One would assume that a statistician available to a medical school, if not to a department of preventive medicine, provides the consultation needed in any academic unit, with or without a consultation program.

While a physician has a wide range of opportunity for consultation and research in preventive medicine, it is important that he concentrate on one or two major areas rather than "dabble" in many of the opportunities provided through the epidemiological approach. This caution is sounded because of the opportunity for a variety of interests. Effective consultation in medical care problems requires a degree of specialization, through training and experience, not unlike specialization in other clinical fields. For example, consultation in medical care systems with corresponding interest in medical education are two fields which, in their interrelationship, provide opportunity for a wide range of study and consultation. The fields of clinical virology, heart disease, mental illness, or malignancy each demand a degree of concentration that would not permit attention to other areas of interest and still yield effective results. Therefore, the physician in the department of preventive medicine, while being in a discipline that has a wide range of possibilities in the application of common denominators of prevention, must in the interest of greatest service and contribution decide upon one major area, or two closely related areas for consultation and research.

The Public Health Nurse

The addition of a public health nurse to the medical school faculty on a full-time academic basis precluded any service responsibility. The focus on comprehensive medical care teaching was the major reason for interest in having a public health nurse available to the department. It was difficult, however, to find a public health nurse interested in a full-time position on a medical school faculty. Current trends in nursing education still separate the physician and nurse educator. There is an increasing tendency for nursing education to be given predominantly by nursing faculty rather than by physicians as was the case a few years ago. Indeed, a staff member of a prominent nursing organization has said that nurses should not participate in medical education because the paths of nurses and physicians educationally are becoming more divergent, and there is less need for physicians to serve as instructors in a nursing education program. There is some reason to doubt that this is entirely the case, since physicians will always be needed to teach, at least in part, some of the basic elements of medicine to a profession that is so closely allied with the technology of medicine.

The first experience in the Vermont program with a full-time public health nurse took place in the development of the Family Care Unit. The particular responsibility of the public health nurse was to function as a liaison between the medical school program and the public health nurses of the community, including school nurses. With this liaison, the full-time public health nurse is in a position to interpret to medical students the best use of nursing agencies in the community, and in turn to interpret to these agencies the educational objectives of nursing in the medical education program. In addition, by making home visits and functioning in the offices of the Family Care Unit, the nurse is in a position to point out to students the expectations that a physician may have with respect to the availability of nursing skills in an ambulatory and home care program. Only a nurse can provide this particular orientation. There is a tendency for the medical student and the house officer to fail to recognize the difference between readily available nursing skills in the hospital and those that can be provided reasonably in the patient's home.

In general, the objectives of the public health nurse in a medical education setting are to assist the medical student to be aware of professional relationships and to understand the role of nursing in a health team; to help the student realize the importance and necessity of keeping detailed nurses' notes in patient records; to reinforce the student's awareness of the importance of individualized medical care; to acquaint the student with certain functions of the nurse, such as routine office procedures, maintenance of drugs and supplies, chaperonage of patients, and the like; and to help the student gain an appreciation of the value and the appropriate use of referrals to community nursing agencies.

The relationship between the student and the nurse as a teacher is a difficult one because of the traditional attitude that the nurse is the handmaiden of the physician and inferior to the physician in professional skill and judgment. From a technological point of view with respect to diagnosis and treatment, the nurse indeed is less skilled. Yet the public health nurse in a teaching setting enables the medical student to appreciate the special skills in observation and in continuing care that the nurse provides, particularly in these days of technological advance when the nurse is much more closely involved in the daily care of the patient.

There is no place in the medical school setting in which the student has an opportunity to understand fully the functions of the nurse. In the Family Care Unit, this opportunity exists in that the nurse on the faculty is in fact teaching and has academic rank in the medical school as a teacher. The nurse, functioning as a teacher, also points out appropriate techniques in office maintenance and procedures, maintains supervision of the student's bags used for house calls, and has responsibility for the office staff nurse. The teaching function of the public health nurse is further exemplified through general office management in collaboration with the physician, the director of the unit.

The public health nurse in the unit participates in seminars as a teacher. Here, with a student nurse and sometimes a student

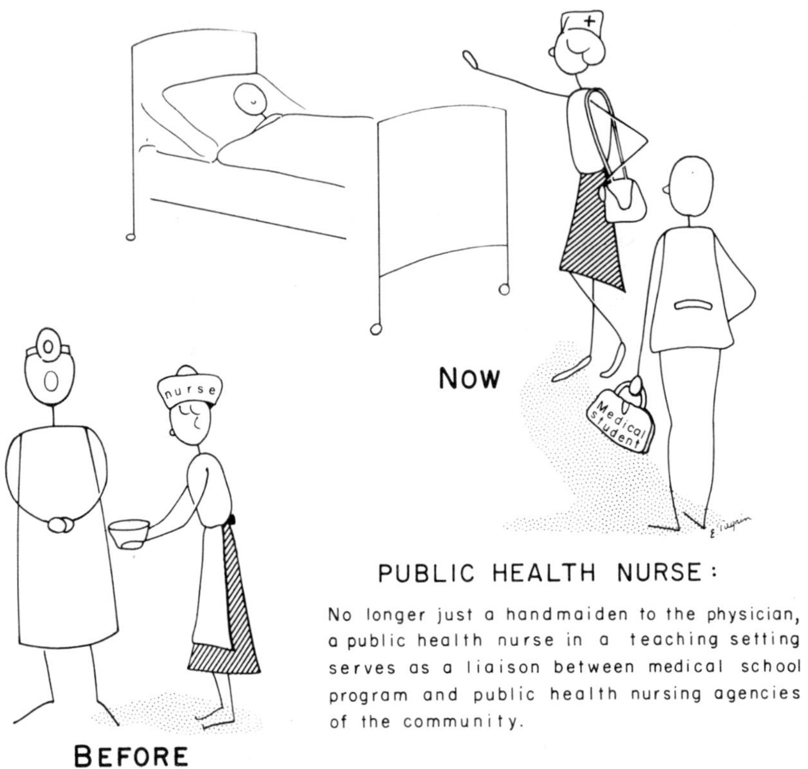

Figure 6

in nutrition present, the public health nurse serves as the guidance director in problems pertaining to the home and family and to public health nursing. Again, the teaching contact is geared to show the students the practical implications for their future practice of medicine.

The public health nurse in the Family Care Unit, as a member of the academic community of the medical school, had a considerably easier role to play than the second public health nurse who came to the department to function primarily in research and to explore teaching on the part of the public health nurse in a hospital setting. Public health nurses in general are not very well prepared for research activity. Consequently, the research in which this public health nurse engaged was primarily directed by team effort and involved such studies as tuberculosis control. The public health nurse did perform a very valuable function as a continuing advisor under my direction in the routine operation of rural health centers. The background and training of public health nurses are such as to enable them to be valuable advisors to trustees of health centers and to physicians inexperienced in the operation of an office.

In the hospital, the public health nurse accompanied physicians on rounds but found it difficult to enter into the situation as a teacher. The public health nurse observed but astutely withheld comments during visits with the patient. She did find increasing opportunities to point out the need for additional information on home situations, the availability of nursing, and the like, prior to the discharge of the patient. A nurse functioning only as a teacher, and without a service component, in the outpatient department of the hospital can make a valuable contribution in the interpretation of demands being made upon the patient and his family, or upon a community nursing agency, in the interim care of the patient. There is much about public health nursing that physicians do not understand, and there is much about public health nursing that students of medicine can and should learn. They should be better equipped to know how to make appropriate use of public health nurses with increasing frequency in their own future practice of medicine.

The exploration of the use of the public health nurse as a teacher in the hospital setting was too brief to warrant any major conclusions. The position of the second public health nurse became vacant, and was not refilled because the financial situation was such as to not warrant expenditure for the purpose of further exploration of the use of the public health nurse as a full-time teacher.

The Health Educator

Health education as a professional discipline has come to be known as an entity unto itself only in the past fifteen years. There has for many, many years been health education as practiced by a variety of individuals including the physician, the nurse, the social worker, the schoolteacher, the chairman of the industrial safety committee, public safety officials, and so on. Today, the health educator, as referred to here, is a person who has come from a variety of backgrounds, including teaching and the biological sciences. With additional graduate training in public health, these individuals have come to be known as health educators in the medical sense.

The health educator in a consultation role has limited opportunity in a department of preventive medicine of a medical school. This is particularly true in situations in which the service role is properly relegated to the service agency, and the medical school is not involved in service.

Utilizing the techniques of health education, the health educator serves a useful function as a member of a team in the

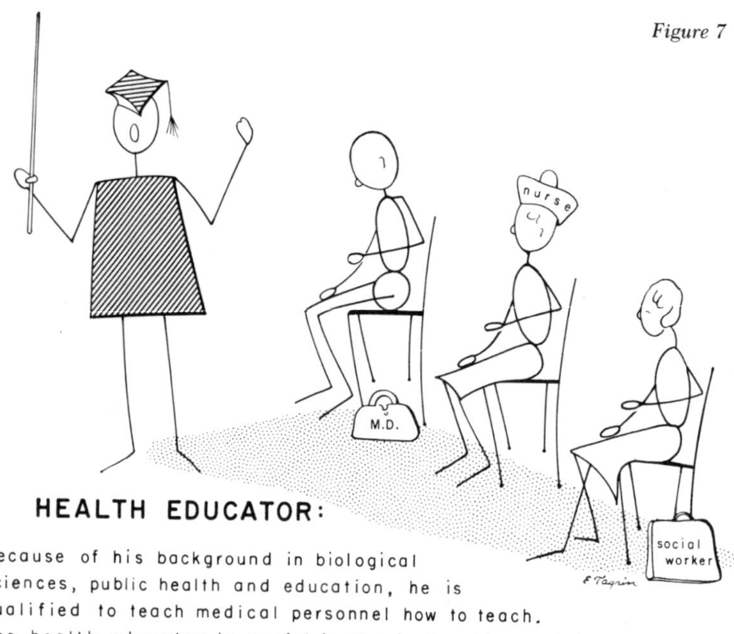

preparation of survey questionnaires. While one might think of the health educator as the individual to serve as the instructor of interviewers for the completion of schedules, this is a role which is hardly so special as to be assigned to any one discipline. Any member of a health team is equipped by professional background to explain a questionnaire to prospective interviewers.

The analysis of various organizations within the context of a regional medical survey is a responsibility which the health educator should be well equipped to discharge. This is particularly true of health education activities of official and voluntary agencies. Yet, one does not assign this type of responsibility as a unique role of the health educator. Almost any member of a team involved in public health or medical care consultation is equipped for such analyses. This is particularly true because of the necessity of having a physician as a member of any such survey team, especially when the survey or consultation has to do with the delivery of medical care or allied services. Otherwise, the team without the physician encounters technical problems that are certain to be raised by either the recipients of medical care or those responsible for delivery of medical care, whether it be a hospital, a community seeking physicians, or a community agency seeking ways and means to improve services. To be sure, the physician may be only a background figure on a team, but without the availability of medical opinion, such surveys would leave much to be desired in completeness of analysis and solution.

The Nutritionist

While students understand the fundamental elements of nutrition through biochemistry, they generally have little opportunity to engage in a teaching session with a dietician. Here, reference is made to the dietician of the hospital, not to the nutritionist. The medical student's experience in the hospital enables him to request therapeutic diets, but usually with little opportunity to discuss the economic and social implications of placing a patient on a particular dietary regime.

To have a nutritionist available on a full-time teaching basis, there must be a research program that will occupy the nutritionist's time when it is not taken up with teaching. The nutritionist in a teaching program in preventive medicine should have some prior experience of working with communities, either through school programs or through public health agencies. While there is some reason to be concerned about the lack of adequate contact between the medical student and the hospital dietician, there is a greater need for the student in a comprehensive medical care program to have an opportunity to discuss the budgetary and social problems of families. Hence, the distinction is made between the dietician and the nutritionist, with emphasis being placed on community and public health aspects of nutrition.

The efforts of the nutritionist during the exploration period were confined almost exclusively to the Family Care Unit. With the nutritionist, as with the public health nurse, emphasis was to be on teaching rather than on service. Service to some extent was provided in the course of making contact with families assigned to medical students to obtain information as to food habits, budgetary limitations, and the like. Perhaps the greatest teaching service rendered by the nutritionist was the development of insight into economic and cultural problems as they relate to difficulties in getting patients to follow a particular dietary regime.

The nutritionist had the opportunity, as did other members of the department, to talk with seniors in the preventive medicine conferences of the fourth year. The time allotted the nutritionist was used both to observe student deficiencies in dealing with problems in nutrition, and to understand the approaches that a nutritionist could use in teaching fourth-year medical students. Here, as was the case in all the teaching situations involving allied health personnel, the student was not particularly interested, unless the approach in teaching gave him some substance of utilitarian value for the practice of medicine.

The opportunity for interdisciplinary effort by the nutritionist, the health educator, and the sociologist occurs frequently. This triad of associated disciplines provides an excellent opportunity for research into the nutritional habits of population groups. As long ago as 1888, Atwater called on social scientists to help explain why the poor considered foods with the most delicate appearance, and the highest price, to be the most desirable.

Points of teaching contact for the nutritionist can extend from the comprehensive medical care program to the outpatient department of the hospital, and into the inpatient services. The nutritionist with a public health background has an orientation to community medicine that the therapeutic dietician of the hospital usually lacks. If there is to be a nutritionist on the faculty, one would do well to consider the assets of a nutritionist with professional advancement that has included experience in research. There is not sufficient demand for teaching time in the medical school curriculum for the nutritionist, or for any professional discipline, to be fully occupied in teaching without additional research or administrative activities.

The faculty in preventive medicine at Vermont no longer includes a full-time nutritionist. It was decided to drop this position, principally because of the relatively small advantage which accrues from having a full-time nutritionist. Ways can be worked out which bring the hospital dietician as a teacher into greater contact with medical students. In a university with a home economics department, there also is the potential for cooperative endeavor between the colleges of the home economics and medicine in sharing the teaching services of a nutritionist. The comprehensive medical care program at Vermont has included, as noted earlier, experience for some students in nutrition as well as for medical students and nurses. There is then ample availability of nutrition teaching through intercollege participation without greatly increasing the cost of medical education, and with the added dividend of increased shared responsibilities among university, colleges and departments.

The Social Scientist

The inclusion of a representative of the behavioral sciences in the developing program at Vermont was dictated by the controversy of the times as to the place of the social scientist in medical education. With a major element of regional consultation into which a sociologist presumably could fit very well, and with the development of a curriculum in preventive medicine, this setting seemed to be particularly suited for testing the abilities of the medical sociologist.

Much has been written about the place of the social scientist in medical education. There is probably greater agreement on the usefulness of the social scientist in research than in any other area of contemplated function. The controversy arises between the utilitarian schools and the schools of thought that find medicine something more than utilitarian. Alcuin, in his "Patrologia Latina," published in 1617, but written about 804 A.D., emphasized the fact that ". . . medicine, like architecture, was not a liberal study which would elevate the mind and lead to thought and contemplation. It was presumably a useful and practical art, like many others" (Selwyn-Brown, 1928).[3]

Then there is the statement, astounding to some, that "medicine is a social science" (Smillie 1955).[4] These pronouncements have varying impact depending upon the orientation of the audience. To those who are geared to the prominence of social science participation in medical education, these emphases sometimes suggest that social science in and of itself comprises medicine. The approach taken in the program at the University of Vermont in the utilization of the sociologist was that medicine is a biological science, but that it is concerned too with behavioral phenomena. On this basis there was ample opportunity for exploration of the medical sociologist's services as a teacher in direct contact with the student, in addition to his participation in the regional program discussed earlier in Part II.

McIntire[5], writing in 1894 in the *Bulletin of the American Academy of Medicine* (now known as the *Journal of Sociological Medicine*), cites the Century Dictionary definition of sociology as: "The science of social phenomena, the science which treats of the general structure of society, the laws of its development, the progress of civilization . . ." And then as to medical sociology, McIntire says that it is: "The science of the social phenomena of the physicians themselves, as a class apart and separate; and the science which investigates the laws regulating the relation between the medical profession and human society as a whole." While one might entertain the idea that medical sociology in fact is as old as McIntire's use of the term, actually McIntire, a physician, was thinking of the social service aspects of medical practice, and was characterizing the physician as a person necessarily concerned with the social welfare of his patients. This is somewhat different from the present connotation of medical sociology.

This term now implies an adjunct discipline allied with the medical profession in teaching and research and, in some quarters, in services as well for the future. Without medical sociology, there would presumably not be comprehensive medical care. This was not the medical sociology of McIntire.

Like the allied health personnel, the medical sociologist accepted appointment in the Department of Preventive Medicine at the University of Vermont with an understanding that the program was to involve both the development of a consultation program to meet the medical needs of the Northeast and an exploration of the potential roles of social science and paramedical personnel in full-time faculty appointments in the medical school. The teaching activities of the sociologist were largely concentrated in the first year. Here the sociologist played a prominent role in setting forth principles of the social aspects of human ecology. In the seminar discussions, there was much opportunity for the sociologist to discuss the application of sociological concepts, largely elementary sociology.

There was some opportunity for the sociologist to work intermittently with the comprehensive medical care program. Of particular interest was a sociological evaluation of the community from which the patient population was coming to the comprehensive medical care program. It became increasingly clear that the sociologist functioned especially well in analysis of community structure, but did not seem to have the appropriate orientation for dealing with practical factors in the application of sociological principles, both in teaching and in research. Throughout the five years there was evidence of difficulty in combining the academic with the practical, and a tendency to denounce practical application as unscholarly. One must admit that there should be a place for the behavioral scientist in the field of medicine, but the traditional training of the sociologist, and special programs to date, have not developed a professional prototype in medical sociology who knows precisely how he can best fit into the picture. This is truer of the social scientist than of paramedical personnel. This is not difficult to understand when one recalls the length of time it has taken the nursing and medical social service professions to develop. The inclusion of the social scientist in a very practical and utilitarian graduate school creates problems as to how he can best meet expectations.

Donald Young, General Director of the Russell Sage Foundation, has commented that: "The collaborating social scientist must know the substantive area of collaboration, not merely his own discipline." This question is pertinent both in teaching and in research in a medical setting. The question is how best to develop the medical sociologist.

Medicine is a profession of many languages. To argue for indoctrination of the social scientist into the language of medicine for ease of communication is to fail to recognize the variety of languages spoken in the medical profession. There is the language of the basic scientist in physiology, biochemistry, and pharmacology. There is the language of the internist, the surgeon, the pathologist, and the pediatrician. It is not a practical goal to attempt to provide orientation in the biological sciences for ease of communication with physicians. The distance is simply too great for the gap to be bridged effectively. For research purposes, the social scientist can receive as much indoctrination as is necessary in much the same manner as does the statistician involved in biological research. In the educational process, it is most desirable that medical students learn to communicate in a language that is understandable to those who have not studied medicine. In the teaching process, it is far better that the medical student understand that the teacher in the behavioral sciences is not a medically trained person and that he must therefore make his technical point clearly so that his teacher in the social sciences can communicate with him. It is courting mediocrity to attempt to develop a technological reference for those who have not spent the requisite time in the premedical and medical aspects of the biological sciences. Requiring the medical sociologist to read a reference library of highly technical journals, audit a few medical lectures, or casually observe an outpatient department or an emergency ward serves only to compound present problems in acceptance of the social scientist in medical teaching and research. Competent clinical and medical administrative guidance must support the social scientist, if there is to be meaningful and reliable participation.

A basic understanding of chemistry, physiology, pathology, and anatomy is necessary for full understanding of the actions, procedures, and reactions of medical personnel. Medical students object when persons with less training than they in the biological sciences presume to make a point in medical practice. The proper training of the social scientist should render him wholly comfortable as a social scientist, and firmly opposed to any attempt to understand the medical process through superficial introduction to it in whatever manner. The delivery of medical care and the reaction between doctor and patient are social phenomena. In this area, the social scientist with particular skills in understanding groups and group reaction, has a contribution to make. Medicine is more than technology. Those who seek to participate in the medical education process must represent a pure discipline without an apparent tendency to usurp, by some superficial understanding, the responsibility vested in the technology of medicine. The biochemist entered the field of medical education as a chemist, without the trappings of medical designators and survey of clinical courses, but with conceptions of the reliability and usefulness of his skills.

The sociologist has innumerable opportunities for participation in research. This is so obvious as to preclude any further comment. The status of long-term illness and the social implications thereof clearly point the way for sociological participation in research. Again, however, the social scientist participating in medical research must remember that research in the medical setting is generally utilitarian in nature, and that the objective of research is to gain information that ultimately can be put to use. There is less opportunity for research that deals with collection and analysis of data only to find out some interesting things in which a few people may have an interest.

In the medical school setting, there are innumerable responsibilities that the sociologist or behavioral scientist might assume. (See Figure 8.) Some may be administrative in nature, such as participation on the library committee, the premedical advisory committee, and the like. The social scientists, however, should adhere carefully to the manner in which they think they can best contribute to teaching and research in a medical setting, rather than leap at every invitation offered them. If they did they would soon find themselves in the position of the nurse and social worker, who only lately are liberating themselves, so to speak, from positions of servitude in order to become truly allied professionals in the provision of medical care.

Medicine as a separate and distinct discipline, wrapped as it

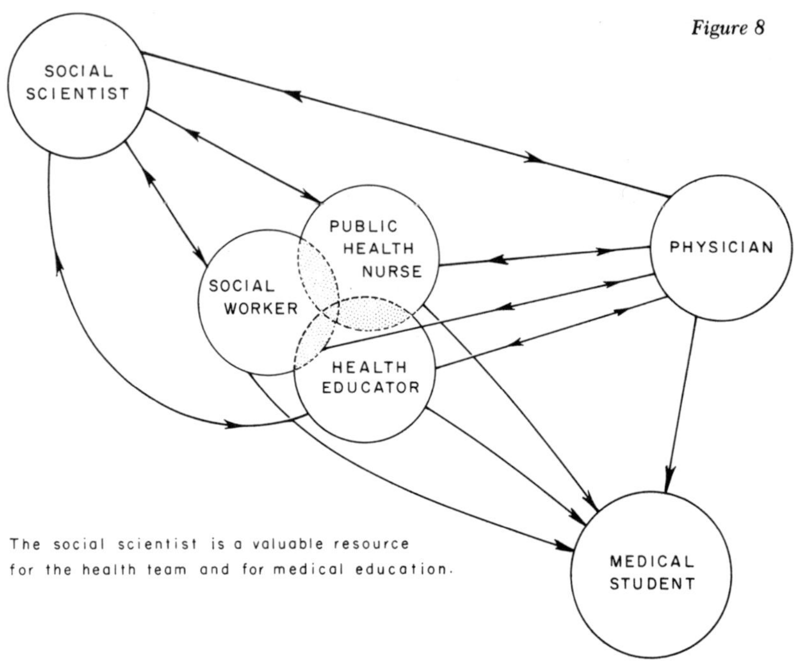

is in deep technology and in the aura of life and death, would benefit much from the objective studies and analyses that social scientists have been able to conduct with ethnic groups, cultural groups, industrial groups, economic groups, and so on. Objective analysis of the practice of medicine or the activities of a section of a hospital, whether it be emergency ward, operating room, or outpatient clinic, can be subject to gross misinterpretation and error, however, if carried out solely by persons lacking knowledge of the basic and clinical sciences. The collaboration of social scientist and physician is essential if the analyses are to be sound.

The association or collaboration of the social scientist with the physician is perhaps most effective in the department of psychiatry, secondly, in the department of preventive medicine, and thirdly in the department of pediatrics or medicine. These are the academic departments in the medical school in which the closest and easiest working relationships between the physician and the social scientist are likely to develop.

The basic years of medical education, commonly referred to as undergraduate medical education, are heavily preoccupied with the development of technological skills. Relatively little time needs to be given to discussion of the concepts of social science. All that is needed is an awareness on the part of the medical student of the relativity of social science and physical science. If students have had a liberal college education, their studies of the medical problems of long-term illness, gerontology, diseases of stress, twentieth-century nutrition, and so on, do not need to be saturated with social science.

In the first half of the twentieth century, the number of physicians increased 60 percent, while the number of personnel engaged in health services increased by at least 400 percent (Orr, 1960)[6]. As yet, social scientists, other than clinical psychologists, are not included generally in the count of personnel engaged in health services. Whether or not they will ever be depends upon the specific professional development of their field as a practical adjunct to the primarily biological concerns of medicine.

The more general acceptance of the social scientist as a colleague in research implies acceptance of a secondary responsibility for teaching in the medical school. The social scientist is likely to argue for responsibility in direct teaching by pointing to the increased number of Ph.D. scientists who are teachers and investigators in medical schools. That there has been a steady increase in the number of teachers without a doctor of medicine degree in the basic sciences is readily apparent. The Council on Medical Education and Hospitals of the American Medical Association reported in 1959 that almost 70 percent of the full-time faculty members in the five major basic sciences do not hold the doctor of medicine degree.

An editorial in the *J.A.M.A.*, Volume 171, No. 11, November 14, 1959, entitled, "Medicine's Growing Dependence on Allied Scientists," points out ways of safeguarding maintenance for the medical student's opportunity to relate the basic science disciplines to current clinical problems, even with a decreasing number of physician teachers in the major basic sciences. The three safeguards cited are: (1) The free interchange and easy communication that generally exist between basic science and clinical faculty; (2) the perceptiveness of students within whose minds the correlation of basic and clinical phenomena ultimately must take place; and (3) the increasing segment of career clinical teachers who have a sound background in one or more of the basic medical sciences as a necessary qualification for their own teaching and research. (For example, the internist today must be something of a biochemist.)

If the social sciences are to make the contribution to medical education that some now claim they can make, particular attention must be paid to the first and second conditions noted above. It has already been emphasized that it is a mistake to attempt to overcome possible problems of communication by turning social scientists into pseudophysicians by superficial exposure to medical terminology and situations. The social scientist should enter the field of medical education with full faith and credit in the contribution that he can clearly make as a social scientist. The fact that this is an endeavor within a well-defined, well-structured, well-established biological science must be understood.

The second condition invokes the necessity that the social scientist, in teaching medical students, give them material that has utilitarian significance for the future.

The third condition will be met ultimately by physician-teachers. As increasing emphasis is placed on the importance of the social and behavioral sciences, it is reasonable to assume that premedical students will gradually cease to concentrate in the biological and physical sciences. Ultimately a generation of physicians will return to medical schools as teachers who have full appreciation for, and the ability to integrate into their teaching, the relatively simple concepts of the behavioral sciences as they relate to the practice of medicine. The current fascination with the inclusion of the behavioral and social sciences in medicine may be short-lived. Social scientists should devote their greatest efforts to the liberal arts colleges, where all college graduates will, hopefully at least, become informed in matters of behavioral science that are not peculiarly restricted to needs in medical education.

The continued relationship of social scientists with medical schools is very likely to be in research on an intercollege basis within the university. There is apparently sufficient substance in the research approach of the social scientist to enable medical scientists to "get their teeth into it." Ethnic differences, attitudinal surveys, and cultural complexities are much more easily translated into research activity for medical faculty than into medical practice for the medical student.

That the sociologist is a theoretician, and is not equipped to function at a practical level in teaching, nor to some extent in applied research, is a reflection of lack of training for practical endeavors. Scholarly research, if it is confined to the artificiality of classroom and library, is not in itself sufficient for practical approaches in a utilitarian field such as medicine.

The position of medical sociologist at Vermont became vacant. Through a cooperative relationship between the College of Medicine and the College of Arts and Sciences, a sociologist and an anthropologist were available to the program on a part-time basis. Experience over a four-year period did not confirm a need for a full-time sociologist in the medical school, discounting the areas of research that could be financed from other than university funds. The cost of maintaining a full-time sociologist as a faculty member is not warranted, in the light of the experiments now taking place in medical schools and the still vague and nebulous bases for active participation in medical school teaching. The contact provided through intercollege cooperation is sufficient in the first year to provide students with an awareness of the important relationships of cultural phenomena to biological phenomena. Further exposure to social science thinking in the comprehensive medical care program is desirable on a case-selected basis, where the sociologist can contribute to the seminar by elucidating the forces affecting the individual, his family, and the community in the provision of medical care services. That there is a behavioral science element in the practice of medicine is not denied. But, a training program in which the social scientist could effectively "put across" the importance of the relationships between behavioral and physical sciences has not developed.

The program at Vermont maintained depth in accordance with its original purpose of teaching continuous and progressive principles of preventive medicine throughout the four years of medical school; there had also been a maintenance of depth in the comprehensive medical care program without the availability of a full-time health educator, nutritionist, and a part-time sociologist. This depth was maintained simply by recognition of pertinent factors by the faculty now participating, including a very competent, general physician who was able to translate for students the essential principles of the behavioral science in their application to office, home, and hospital practice. Consequently, the program at Vermont continued to direct its efforts toward the teaching of comprehensive medical care, and toward the continuous and progressive development of preventive medicine principles, including the social science point of view, without the undue financial burden of such a heavy staff. Research continued to develop through the joint participation of personnel in the Department of Preventive Medicine, other departments in the medical school, and departments of the other colleges that are interested in related subjects. Likewise, personnel of the Department of Preventive Medicine would always have an interest in participating in research that may be initiated by other departments of the medical school, or by other colleges of the university.

The Medical Social Worker

> While in my bed I lie all day,
> In pain that will not pass away,
> The neighbors come and go. Ah!
> If with them my sweetheart came,
> The doctors would be put to shame:
> She understands my woe!

> —Egyptian lyric poem

That the social conditions of patients are important to diagnosis, treatment, and prognosis has long been recognized by the medical profession. Recognition of environmental factors as important to total understanding of the patient and his family is not new.

In 1913 Dr. David L. Edsall called upon Miss Ida Cannon, director of the social service department of the Massachusetts General Hospital, to assist in a series of lectures to medical students. The story of the establishment of medical social service at the Massachusetts General Hospital by the great Dr. Richard Cabot is too well known to need repetition here.

In 1932 the Commission on Medical Education of the Association of American Medical Colleges took an official stand emphasizing the importance of the social worker to the physician in the provision of comprehensive medical care. In 1939 a study by the Education Committee of the American Association of Medical Social Workers, covering a ten-year period, was published. Miss Marian Russell, director of the Department of Social Services of Montefiore Hospital, was chairman of a study of the teaching responsibility of social workers in medical education. This analysis of participation on the part of social workers, and projected improvement in their teaching and research responsibilities, provided interesting data.

At the peak of development of the Vermont program, two medical social workers were on the staff of the Department of Preventive Medicine. The second social worker was needed in the development of the comprehensive medical care program. The participation of one social worker in research, in teaching, and in the regional program (Part II) demanded the second medical social worker for the exploration phase.

The social worker participated in the teaching of human ecology, both in the orientation phase and in the seminars. Here the social worker had an opportunity to introduce to students who were only one year out of college and in their first year of medicine, the applicability of an understanding of community resources to the practice of medicine. In addition, there was opportunity to present the philosophy of the social worker in dealing objectively with social stress and strain, and not merely functioning as a "do-gooder" in the community.

An introductory lecture to social service, an outline of its history, and the application of social work in a case-method example, was given to second-year students during the time allotted to teaching of medical care systems.

In the third and fourth years, the medical social worker participated fully as a faculty member in the Family Care Unit. In this setting the social worker demonstrated the manner in which a social worker would function on referral of a social problem, and the manner in which the physician would function, if he did not have readily available to him community resources comprising the specialties of social service. Opportunity was taken to point out

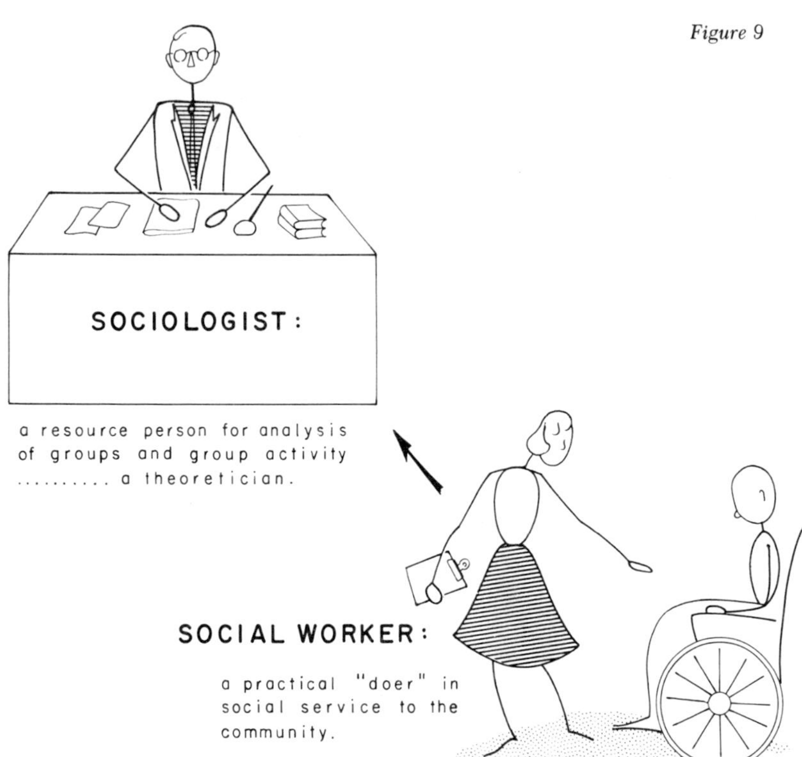

the social service assets vested in the public health nurse, the clergyman, and friends and relatives of the patient in resolving social pathology pertinent to completely definitive care.

The social worker functioned importantly in the teaching of gerontology. This was a senior-year experience in which the student was assigned to one resident of a home for the aged operated in affiliation with one of the teaching hospitals.

Later, there was one medical social worker on a full-time basis in the Department of Preventive Medicine. There was no need to "gild the lily" in efforts to demonstrate that a medical school is riding the frontiers of progressive and advancing medical education. That this pertinent concept can be gotten across to the students and depth of meaningful program maintained are the important factors. Without at least one full-time medical social worker, however, no program can teach comprehensive medical care as a basis for demonstrating the fusion of clinical and preventive medicine.

Early in the days at Vermont, I visited the institutions affiliated with the medical school. These consisted of state and federal hospitals and voluntary community hospitals. In order to extend the principles of preventive medicine teaching to these affiliated services, a method was sought to bring together those forces that could be utilized in the affiliating institutions in order to have consistency of program wherever the student went. To this end, I encouraged the medical social worker to meet with the social workers in these affiliated institutions. Out of this association of social workers, employed in institutions in which medical students receive clinical experience, came an informal organization known as the "Social Workers Participating in Medical Education." A full-time medical social worker with the Department of Preventive Medicine submitted a description of this voluntary teaching association for publication in the *Journal of Social Work*.

The group of social workers involved in this teaching association included those from voluntary and official agencies such as an institution for unwed mothers, a crippled children's service, social service departments of hospitals, a rehabilitation center, a mental hospital, a children's rehabilitation center, and a sectarian social agency. The objectives of this group of social workers in meeting voluntarily with a full-time medical social worker on the faculty of the medical school were:

1. To clarify the role of the social worker in the case setting.

2. To orient the student to the setting with its particular health and social problems.

3. To interpret community health and welfare resources to the students, and to explain how to refer a patient to such resources.

4. To help the students to understand the nature of social and health problems.

5. To develop students' sensitivity to social and emotional problems.

6. To help students define joint areas of action for the physician and the social worker.

7. To support the student in times of stress in his doctor-patient relationship.

8. To interpret the solution to problems worked out by other social agencies, especially when they may not be consistent with the student's thinking.

9. To help students understand the emotional aspects of illness.

10. To assist, whenever possible, in matters of interviewing.

While there might be some justification for having a social worker available in all of the teaching settings in which the medical student finds himself, this would be neither administratively nor financially feasible for most medical schools. There must be at least one full-time medical social worker in an academic capacity if adequate time is to be given to the teaching of comprehensive medical care. To bridge the gap between the need for and the availability of social workers, and in recognition of the profession's natural desire to teach whenever the opportunity presents itself, bringing a group of social workers engaged in service into the academic atmosphere via the full-time social worker is apparently both practical and stimulating. The social workers function better as teachers in their contacts with medical students when they render service in whatever medical or social setting the student may occupy.

One cannot envision how the medical student can develop understanding of comprehensive medical care unless he has an opportunity to understand community resources, including the criteria for effective social service, through adequate academic and practical experience. The usefulness of social work, like the usefulness of nursing, is usually so obvious to the medical student as not to require much examination in the teaching program. The need to interpret and to reinterpret the applicability of social science, health education, and nutrition arises from the deficiency in training background of these disciplines for participation in medical education.

In addition to the usual interpretation of social services in comprehensive medical care the social worker could make a potentially great contribution in interviewing. Social workers have unusual skill in the interview technique, both in the interview situation itself and as interpreters of the significance of the replies and comments of interviewees. While no direct attempt has been made to utilize the social worker in this capacity in teaching, it is readily apparent from experience, particularly in the Family Care Unit, that the interview technique should be taught by a person skilled in social work. This could be included in the second year, when the student is taught how to elicit data as a part of his course in physical diagnosis.

The Statistician

The importance of a statistician to adequate research programs is so obvious as not to merit extended discussion.

The teaching of biometrics and vital statistics to medical students is under constant discussion, and there are many obvious ways in which this teaching can be done. In teaching vital statistics and biometrics, one must take into consideration the block that so many medical students seem to have concerning mathematics. To gain their confidence early in the presentation of statistical methods one can simply use a well-known technique for dealing with any subject matter they find difficult to accept. The plan is to increase the time given to the teaching of applied medical statistics (vital statistics and biometrics) by inclusion of some hours in the first year, with more time to relate applied medical statistics to second-year teaching, particularly to epidemiology, and hopefully, to the third- and fourth-year teaching in the Family Care Unit. At the present time, there is an opportunity only to present some basic principles of biometrics. The main objective in teaching biometrics to medical students is to equip them for intelligent reading of scientific journals. This does not require that a medical student become highly proficient in the use of statistics.

The fact that the statistician has basic training in one major field, and must become familiar with a second field in order to function as a consultant in research design and analyses in medicine, is a factor that applies to all paramedical and social science personnel who participate in medical education. The statistician who knows the field of biometrics well seeks other professional guidance in the execution of statistical design and analysis. This course should be followed by all paramedical and social science personnel who strive to function in the medical education process.

Interdisciplinary Relationships

In a program as broadly conceived as that developed at Vermont, serious consideration had to be given to the interrelationship of these disciplines and to the manner and the substance of the contribution that each might make. It was important that each discipline test objectively how it might contribute to the modification of medical education for tomorrow's needs, not engage in a struggle with other professional disciplines over which might be most important to the cause. The human trait of egocentrism is just as applicable to professional disciplines as it is to individuals.

It was assumed that if a professional person were given ample opportunity to discover areas of application in which he might apply his own field in a new setting, a lively, well-balanced program would be more likely to result. That such freedom led to a lively program is without question, and development of the curriculum testifies to the fact that a balanced program was achieved as a result of the participation of a variety of professional disciplines. Nevertheless, as was noted previously, the maintenance of a program in depth in a department of preventive medicine does not require the full-time presence of all of the possible disciplines that could be of importance in one way or another.

As each representative of these various disciplines joined the program, time was allowed for orientation to the local situation and for appreciation of the philosophy under which the program was being launched. The orientation period also permitted the members of the department to become acquainted personally and professionally, and enhanced their understanding of their separate responsibilities by virtue of their professional training and by experience. New personnel must be guided, but in such a way as to give them a freedom of action commensurate with the need to pool independent professional thinking to derive the maximum benefit possible from cooperative endeavor. Understanding and determined application, coupled with enthusiasm and sincerity of purpose, are the essential ingredients for molding a staff into a program in preventive medicine that is certain to deliver findings of interest in the academic field. If such a program reaches its full potential, it extends its influence through the medical school into other departments without undue pragmatism.

In addition to orientation to the projected program for development of a department over a period of four to five years, the staff was encouraged to visit throughout the medical school and university, making contacts of interest to their own particular disciplines, and to visit community agencies. Thus the health educator would visit the College of Education; the social worker and the sociologist, the Department of Sociology and the appropriate divisions of the State Health Department; the public health nurse would contact the Department of Nursing of the university and appropriate agencies, and so on.

Staff members were always encouraged to express their opinions freely. This was essential to the development of a department which was concerned with exploring the attitudes, thinking, and orientation of a variety of professional people both in relation to teaching and in relation to the projected consultation program in the region. To encourage the frank expression of opinion is, of course, to invite strains of leadership that might not otherwise exist. The free expression of opinion destroys any insulation the administrator or director may enjoy, and creates a climate in which dynamic group action and interaction come clearly to the fore. To separate personality traits and prejudices from professional insight and points of view is not difficult over a period of time in an intensive, close-working relationship. In this intimate atmosphere, as the interprofessional roles developed, it became clear that the directors had to work constantly with the staff in order to maintain feelings of equity as to responsibility, need, and importance in the program. It was especially important that one professional discipline did not set itself up as consultant to other professional disciplines within the department, or in working relationships to each other outside the department. Use of this terminology in relation to other members of the group implies something greater in wisdom and contributory power, and if continued, would adversely affect the contributions of the rest of the team.

These comments on interprofessional relationships result from intensive associations with several disciplines in a program that had, as its stated purpose, arriving at some impressions as to the usefulness of these several disciplines in the medical school setting. The comments in this section are not based on anything other than impressions. There is some time to go yet before any definitive statement can be made with respect to the appropriate roles of social scientists and various paramedical personnel in medical schools.

One early observation, sustained throughout the experience, concerned acceptance of social scientists and paramedical personnel by medical students and faculty alike. It was repeatedly proved that disciplines such as nursing and medical social service, which offer something specific and useful for medical action, were more readily accepted by both medical student and faculty. That some medical faculty believe themselves fully competent to provide social service to patients in the course of providing technical medical care is an attitude that will continue for some time to come. The nature of the profession has imbued the practitioner with the conviction that he is providing social service to his patients when they need it.

The acceptance of nursing in medical school teaching is limited by the traditional view of the nurse as assistant to the physician. The relationship between the physician and the nurse must never be such that the nurse feels free to assume responsibility in technical areas in which she has not been trained. The ambivalent status of the teaching nurse—on the one hand a subsidiary in the delivery of medical care, and on the other hand a teacher of medical students—places the nurse in a difficult position, particularly if her faculty position carries no service identification. Even though achieving acceptance of the nurse as a teacher without a service function will be a slow, difficult process, the nurse's situation is still much easier than those of representatives of disciplines that are relatively new to the medical school, particularly health education and social science. The medical social worker and the public health nurse enjoy, as a result of the historical development of their professional roles, acceptance within the medical setting as professionals with a basic and legitimate interest in medical care and medical education. No accusation of idle curiosity can be lodged against them. Their professional backgrounds and capabilities tend to remove this barrier to the development of teaching responsibilities in the medical setting. The language of the nurse and of the medical social worker is readily understandable to physicians.

The sociologist and the social worker have problems in their medical school relationships principally because of the theoretical background of the former and the practical orientation of the latter. The social worker is of necessity interested in "getting things done," in resolving problems, and in taking action. The sociologist, on the other hand, has a tendency to theorize about behavior in the community or in the neighborhood, but is not equipped in his professional training to take action. But as a resource person in community analysis and the like, the sociologist makes a unique contribution to the social worker, to the public health nurse, and to the health educator.

The health educator should be particularly well equipped to place emphasis on health education through a strong background in education per se. The health educator could profitably be used both in the development of better educational techniques and in a teaching setting in both the inpatient and outpatient services of the hospital. In these situations the health educator is relating closely to the public health nurse, and to some extent to the medical social worker, but more particularly to the former.

The health educator and the nutritionist have much in common because of the importance of didactic teaching in nutrition. As with the other disciplines, there is need to use appropriate educational techniques in order to change attitudes and to effect desired action. The nutritionist needs the assets of a more structured understanding of functions of community, community groups, neighborhoods, and the like that the sociologist can contribute.

The responsibilities of the social worker and the public health nurse overlap to a great extent. Both are in frequent contact with families, and both are in intimate contact with social situations affecting health and recovery from illness. The social worker has a greater skill in analysis of social pathology than does the public health nurse, and naturally has a more informed approach to the solution of social problems. There is an asset that the social worker and public health nurse can bring to the medical student as he observes their different approaches to problems, and has an opportunity to discuss with them both individually and in seminar the problems of patients and their families. In teaching medical students, the social worker can point out that the public health nurse can be utilized as a generalist in meeting challenges of comprehensive medical care when the skills of a social worker are not available.

Because most medical students see medicine as consisting only of diagnosis and treatment, they are more likely to give credence to teaching by a nonphysician if a physician is in attendance, either as a direct participant or as an observer, whether in lecture or in seminar where the nonmedical staff teaches. This is not intended to denigrate the contribution that can be made by these professionals, nor to suggest that they need supervision in the delivery of a lecture or in the conduct of a seminar. It simply recognizes, and attempts to overcome, the fact that medical students (and some faculty members) do not yet accept unquestionably the place of these disciplines in medical school teaching. It is far better to work with a few classes in the gradual introduction of these disciplines foreign to the thinking of the medical student, than to force his indulgence.

Observations over the five-year period clearly indicate that the most effective current roles for the sociologist, the health educator and the statistician are as resource persons to other faculty. Their participation in research can be collaborative or independent.

The nutritionist has a direct teaching opportunity in emphasis on public health nutrition, dealing with economics in home management as well as with the specifics of therapeutic dietetics. In this manner the public health nutritionist can supplement, in an ambulatory medical care program, the therapeutic dietetics that the student may encounter in his hospital experience.

The public health nurse and the social worker have a distinct teaching role in a curriculum that stresses comprehensive medical care. These two professional disciplines now have something definite and utilitarian for the practice of medicine to present to the student.

These comments citing the contributions that can be made by the several allied professional disciplines to medical education and medical research are not, however, automatic endorsement of the representation of all of the disciplines on the medical school faculty. This conclusion is not supported by five years of intensive experience. In the true perspective of university effort, administrative lines separating colleges by reason of major interest or special purpose should be so flexible as to make possible intercollege participation in the service both of improved educational method and of economy. Flexibility in intercollege relationships would create opportunities for greater diversification in educational method and in the scope of research activity that could take place. Experiments in specialized education can take place between colleges.

The members of only four disciplines are seen as essential to the full development of the principles of preventive medicine teaching in the medical school. These four are the physician, the nurse, the social worker, and the statistician. The statistician need not be a full-time member of the department of preventive medicine, but his availability encourages depth of research as well as frequency of research projects, leading to conclusions in a reasonable period of time with periodic published progress reports. If no statistician is available, such criteria for progressive research are likely not to be met, and much valuable time may well be wasted because of poor research design.

The number of physicians in the department of preventive medicine will depend upon the program. At the University of Vermont the focus was on the development of programs of consultation on medical care to a region, with particular emphasis on rural medical needs, and of comprehensive medical care teaching. For each of these programs one full-time physician was needed. Moreover, the development of research in fields other than medical care and allied areas of interest demanded the presence of a physician skilled in research, particularly in clinical virology. The preventive medicine program at the University of Vermont therefore commanded the full-time availability of three physicians. There are, in addition, nine part-time physicians who assist in carrying out the teaching program. These did not include the physician who, on a part-time basis, headed the Division of Rehabilitation, and the physician to be appointed on a part-time basis to head the Division of Occupational Medicine when it is fully developed.

The social scientist, the health educator, and the nutritionist can be adequately available through intercollege effort. Representatives of other disciplines in the university complex ought to be brought into the medical school, at least on a brief-exposure basis. These include experts in political science, economics, and history.

Implications for Curricula in Graduate Schools

While we discuss the student of medicine and approaches to be taken in educational programs, there is as great a question concerning the kinds of teachers that will be needed. My experience in medical administration, and in medical education, has made me curious, too, about the curricula of graduate professional schools.

The following comments are only impressions gained from intensive work with a variety of personnel over the past five years, reinforced by discussions I had had in the course of visits to various schools of public health, schools of social work, schools of medicine, and to some departments of social science in universities. Gradually, and haltingly, steps are being taken toward the achievement of ideals in medical education and in graduate schools for the development of professional individuals who will take their places in both the service and the educational fields. It is not too early to think boldly and to act boldly in the establishment of educational programs that will bring forth persons appropriately prepared for the problems of the decades ahead.

The school of public health is traditionally the fountainhead of preparation in both preventive medicine and public health for physicians and allied professions. It is in the university with a complex of colleges, including a school of public health, that one can best see the potentialities for curricula rearrangement directed at practical preparation for work in the field, whether it be

160

medical education, industry, or a service agency. These comments are admittedly made without a careful study and review of all that is contained in the present curricula of the various professional schools.

Exploration of the use of social science and paramedical personnel in a medical school setting has led me to the firm conclusion that the graduate schools for training in the variety of professions associated in the total complex of medical care should be unified under a system of total university endeavor. That the associated professionals can contribute to the educational process in medicine cannot be denied by anyone who recognizes the importance of a more comprehensive understanding of man by those responsible for medical and social welfare. At the present time, medical educators who wish to utilize the services of social scientists and paramedical personnel must spend a great deal of time in guidance to help them make practical contributions. These allied professionals can be most useful when the maintenance of an acceptable academic standard goes hand-in-hand with a contribution of utilitarian value.

Universities that have a complex of colleges hold the key to the intercollege educational activity that will prepare today the leaders for tomorrow's efforts in an ever-advancing front of community* and environmental medicine.

The importance of erasing and indeed the necessity of removing rigid administrative lines between colleges and to establish fluid lines of unified purpose in intercollege effort is already recognized in some quarters. The joint enterprise at Western Reserve University in an educational program for the health professions was a major step in the desirable direction of joining educational efforts into a mosaic deliberately designed for improved education and improved service by tomorrow's scientists. There remains the need to give the academic recognition on the basis of merit to allied professionals contributing to education as is now given basic scientists and physicians on medical school faculties.

Perhaps one of the reasons that the usefulness of allied professionals in medical education is being explored without their being granted commensurate academic rank is a feeling that they

---

*Early recognition of a field to become known as "community medicine."

are not now adequately prepared for careers in medical education. For example, while a social worker may be an assistant or associate professor of social work in a college of social work, that person may be only an "associate" in the college of medicine—a rating that has no academic significance. Medical students are generally keen in their perception of symbolism. To use a nurse, a social worker, or a health educator in the teaching program without granting them the academic rank their educational attainments and experience warrant is to say to these medical students, "We feel that paramedical personnel have something to offer to medical education, but not enough to warrant academic status equal to that of the basic scientists and clinicians on a medical school faculty."

Graduate training for participation in medical education carries a common denominator for all potential participants in this field—exposure to courses in education that give a background in the techniques and psychology of education. Everyone participating in medical education, including the physician, should have this element of formal training. Even those in the medical service field who do not engage in teaching of research need to understand the teaching and learning process in the execution of their responsibilities in service agencies. The nurse, the social worker, and the physician constantly need "to teach," since teaching may occur in the course of service to individuals, families or social groups, or in the course of program development and planning for official groups.

A second factor that should be a common denominator to all teachers is an understanding of the research method. Physicians, nurses, social workers, health educators, and nutritionists should have sufficient background in research to be able to function comfortably in an academic setting. Those who do not obtain or seek positions in academic settings can still, if they are research oriented, do much to initiate important research in a service agency that can be carried on in conjunction with its public service. If necessary, research in the agencies could be carried out in conjunction with nearby universities, particularly in cases where those employed by the agencies have no time to conduct the research themselves.

The health educator, like the public health nurse and medical social worker, needs to be familiar with the implications of particular diagnoses in order to function well. And, to function comfortably in patient and family contact, he must be competent to take the lead in individual and in group health education. The health educator should therefore have training in bacteriology and modified courses in anatomy and physiology. The health educator must be the type of person, however, who can comfortably regard this material as background reference. He should not be tempted to see himself as virtually a physician. The extent to which the health educator studies biological sciences is a matter that can be decided between the school of public health, and school of medicine, and the school of education. In the training program for health education, these three colleges must have a functional relationship with one another, the college of education taking the lead and the school of public health and the medical school functioning as complementary and supplementary resources.

The health educator with this kind of technical background will be in the position of the statistician in that he has to borrow from other fields, receive indoctrination as to the particular problems at hand, and then proceed to teach or to give consultation based on the problem presented.

If these requirements for the competent health educator are accepted, it is evident that the graduate program for health education should be lengthened to two years. The health educator may be recruited as a college student, and through appropriate educational counseling, led through a continuum of professional preparation beginning early in a collegiate career and terminating in the tripartite effort of the college of education, the school of public health, and the medical school.

The public health nurse is already receiving graduate experience in schools of public health or in schools of nursing. Like the physician in preventive medicine, the nurse, to be acceptable to students and colleagues alike, must have clinical competency in public health. Even with this, the traditional subsidiary role of the nurse will for another generation or longer bar the realization of a true teacher relationship between nurse and medical student. This is unfortunately true, even though medical students absorb from nurses a tremendous amount of valuable orientation, information, and techniques as clinical clerks in their hospital assignments.

In the development of the public health nurse, the common

denominators noted above for all professions allied with medicine are equally applicable. Even though the nurse should have increased opportunity for a role in teaching, the important traditional relationship in which the nurse responds to the physician's directions in diagnosis and treatment must be maintained. Nevertheless, the public health nurse, as well as other members of the health team, must make frank and original contributions if both are to derive the greatest benefit from the multidisciplinary approach in medical education. The nurse's obligation to obey the physician's instructions can be maintained even when the nurse assumes, on the one hand, the role of teacher, and on the other hand, the role of assistant to the physician in the delivery of medical care. The inclusion of medical students, student nurses, and students of nutrition in the same teaching program has long-range implications for the development of future professional relationships among the members of the health team that will lead to genuine comprehensiveness of care with the pooling of original and frank professional opinion. When pointing out the contribution that the nurse can make as a teacher, one must also call attention to the fact that the physician must accept the nurse as a partner on the team without relinquishing his control of the medical situation. Only the physician who has met the requirements in the basic and clinical sciences is competent to diagnose, to initiate treatment; modify or terminate treatment; and to assume full professional and legal responsibility for patients and their families. The full acceptance of the nurse as a bona fide member of the teaching team will come as some nurses accept the challenge to move boldly into new areas in spite of the difficulties they will encounter. Like coral, this structural design will have to be built up one layer at a time.

There is much interest in the appropriate preparation of the social scientist for a role in medical education, and to some extent, in medical research. Porterfield (1960)[7] points out that the two streams of medical and social knowledge have been flowing separately for too long. It is his supposition that each stream by itself cannot fully meet the problems of health maintenance, and he further suggests that ". . . social knowledge is the only medium by which it will be possible to understand the variable meanings of sickness and health in persons; what sick and well persons mean to their families; why families respond to afflicted members as they do; and how families culturally define values, and the responses of others to patients become factors in making people sick, helping them to get well, and motivating them to stay well." The soundness of this point of view can hardly be doubted.

The problem is one of professional preparation for a role in medical education and in medical research that will enable the social scientist to function on a practical as well as a theoretical level. Philosophers can do much to influence the thinking and to modify the actions of some population groups, but those who are engaged in medical activity must have an appropriate professional development, if their points of view, attitudes, and approaches are to be truly useful. The whole problem with the social scientist is that one does not know just how to use him. And the reason that it is difficult to know how to use the social scientist is the fact that so far no one has hit upon the best way to prepare him for a practical function in medical activity. The demand which some medical schools have made for social scientists, and the tremendous competition involving unreasonable levels of salary, have sharpened the problem.

There is general agreement among leading educators in the fields of medicine and public health that the social scientist is yet "not ready" to participate in medical school teaching. Consequently many schools have not attempted to use the social scientist in direct teaching, except in a conference setting in which a physician, and possibly other members of a health team, are present. Until there is high-level agreement between the Council on Medical Education of the American Medical Association and the Association of American Medical Colleges and the several associations of behavioral scientists, there can be no firm and effective solution to the problem of adequate and suitable preparation of the social scientist for participation in the medical field. The social scientist as yet doesn't really know how to function in medical education.

The argument that social scientists should be exposed to medical technology so that they may communicate more easily with medical students and thus teach more effectively is fallacious. It is far better that the medical student be forced to explain himself clearly to the nonmedically trained individual. Contact with nonmedically trained teachers is good for the medical student, particularly if it requires that he put what he means with respect to organic difficulties involving the patient or the family into clear English.

The social scientist interested in the medical scene should have an opportunity to work with hospitals and medical schools that will be critical of his endeavors during his graduate training. The social scientist needs to have experience delivering a finished project on time and with specific recommendations for action. Some sociologists in the field have, over a period of years, learned how to function in a medical setting, and have come to appreciate that their contribution must be practical to be of value in medical education and research. They have not been through any formal program of training, but have learned, through their own astute observations and critical self-assessment of their professional capabilities, to function efficiently in the university complex with particular interests in medical and allied fields.

There is no particular need to designate the sociologist as a "medical" sociologist. His contribution as a sociologist is the important thing, and the prefix "medical" denotes a technical orientation which the social scientist does not and would not have without several more years of hard technical work. After all, it is becoming more and more common for the medical social worker to be known simply as the social worker.

The educational program for the sociologist who aspires to involvement in medical education or medical research should be such as to enable him to see his professional activity in its proper perspective. The social scientist is not likely to have a service role like that of the nurse, the social worker, or the nutritionist.

The greatest professional and educational service social scientists could render to the medical field today is to enter into discussions with the Association of American Medical Colleges and the Council on Medical Education of the American Medical Association concerning the program that might best prepare the social scientist for his particular role in medical education.* This action would help immeasurably to develop a training program that

*Hollingshead at Yale has done much in this direction.

would equip the social scientist to function practically as well as theoretically in the medical setting. Such discussions could lead to the establishment not only of criteria for programs of graduate training for social scientists, but also of criteria for the admission of these professional groups to the field of medical education and research.

The school of public health, because of its long experience in the development of a variety of professional personnel, would be an ideal partner in the training of the social scientist for participation in the medical field. The school of public health, the college of education and the department of social sciences of the university together could fuse their efforts in a coordinated program of training for the social scientist.

The social worker usually comes to the medical school with a good deal of experience with medical problems. The school of public health has much to offer the social worker by serving as the coordinator between the major school of emphasis—the school of social work—and the school of education.

For social workers, and the members of other disciplines, the school of public health should continually provide summer institutes of six to eight weeks, designed as "refresher courses." Those who have been fully occupied in professional work for some time would welcome the opportunity to "catch up" with the thinking and the trends of the times. Intensive institutes at regularly occurring intervals for all health workers should be taking place in schools of public health, as are summer institutes in the physical sciences. Only a university with colleges of medicine, public health, and education, and with strong departments of social sciences, would be in a position to offer coordinated professional graduate training programs, and summer refresher courses, to the wide range of professional groups involved in preventive medicine and public health.

The American dream of peak efficiency in promoting health and lengthening the span of active life is practicable. The contributions in the social sciences and the physical sciences of many universities have been great. I would plead for a welding of inter-college effort in order to promote greater efficiency and greater promise for the achievement of goals and the solutions of problems in the decades ahead.

F

Relationship of the Consulting
University to a State Health Department

While state universities have no monopoly on a potential consultation service to either a state or a given region, certainly they have a definite obligation imposed upon them either implicitly or expressly by the state legislature to perform a specific service or services to the state in addition to that of granting various academic degrees.

While consideration here is given to the relationship of the consulting university to the state health department, such a consulting responsibility could extend to the local or county health departments as well. In Vermont and in New Hampshire local and county or district health departments are conspicuous by their absence. There are organized local and district health departments in Maine. The establishment of working relationships would in any case start with discussion at a mutual level of responsibility, namely between the university and the state health department, with progressive consultation to the local, district, or county level. There is, in fact, much that the consulting university could do to initiate and promote the establishment of local health departments. Where the need is obvious, or in situations where an appropriate survey for local governmental units suggests the establishment of a local or district health department, an agency other than the state health department might be more effective in promoting such thinking. People are innately suspicious! In one of the activities of the Regional Medical Needs Program, the Department of Preventive Medicine met with a committee formed principally by the Vermont Tuberculosis and Health Association, in discussions concerning the establishment of local or district health departments for the State of Vermont. At that time it was provident to concur in the opinion of the majority of the committee that local and district health departments should not be established because the state health department was then sufficiently available to a small population (378,000) distributed over readily accessible territory. It was agreed that what was needed for an overall improvement of public health services in the state was additional personnel to improve the ratio of public health personnel to population. It was decided, however, that it would be desirable to establish at least one autonomous local health unit as a demonstration, with the Burlington area selected as the logical site because of the presence of the medical school and the teaching hospitals there.

Section 1 of the 1949 Public Health Acts of the State of Vermont, No. 184, approved as of July 1, 1949, states in part that the department of health is created ". . . to promote a strong, active coordinated health program." This provision clearly indicates the desirability of the state health department participating with the state medical education institution in activity that would lead to "a strong, active, coordinated health program." Not only does such a provision imply desirable coordination and cooperation with the state medical institution, but it also implies cooperation with other departments of the university which in their educational, research, or consultation programs would be of material interest and benefit to the health and well-being of the people of the state. Specifically, the Vermont statutes provide that the University of Vermont, College of Medicine, cooperate with rural communities in procuring the services of physicians "and other medical *needs* . . . and the prosecution of research into the cause, prevention, and control of disease." Certainly the prosecution of research into the causes, prevention, and control of disease does not confine itself to research in the biological laboratory. One readily recognizes the complementary relationship of community research and laboratory research.

With respect to the responsibility of the university in assisting with the availability of paramedical personnel, section 481 of chapter 212 of the Public Law Acts specifies that "the moneys annually appropriated in favor of the College of Medicine of the University of Vermont shall be used for the purpose of establishing in connection with the College of Medicine a department to be organized for the purpose of cooperating with the rural communities in aiding such communities in procuring physicians and *nurses*." (Italics added.) This dictum gave a legal basis for the establishment of a consultation service extended into the state by a department within a medical school.

Two major conclusions were drawn after review of the legislation. First, the state health department, by law, is the major but not the sole state agency authorized to provide public health services to the state. Secondly, the enabling acts for the establishment of public health clearly point the way for cooperative endeavor in establishing a "strong, active coordinated health program." Thirdly, there is, at least by implication, a substantial interest in the training of public health nurses as imposed under the responsibility of the health commission. In the State of Vermont this interest in the training of public health nurses would logically involve cooperative endeavor with the Department of Nursing in the College of Education.* The statutes relating to the College of Medicine give it the responsibility for rural medical care evaluation, planning, and implementation to meet the medical needs of rural communities. With respect to the "prosecution of research into the cause, prevention, and control of disease," however, there is clearly an area of possible conflict between the state university and the State Department of Health.

Since desirable attitudes and action cannot be legislated, it was and is necessary to cooperate with the state health department, and to show willingness to keep it fully informed concerning the development of the Department of Preventive Medicine, and particularly its extramural activities. Insistence on legal rights can help solve some situations, but it is certainly a mechanism of low priority in the development of any regional plan. An agency

*Now the Rowell College of Allied Health Sciences (1972).

can also fail to meet its full obligation to the public by resorting to the literal interpretation of the "laws on the books."

The department's approach, then, was to forget about its legal justification for establishing a program, and instead to attempt to engage the interest of an agency by open and voluntary discussion of philosophy and plans. In the development of the program at Vermont, I made its purpose as clear as I could in the time available. On two different occasions I had the opportunity to discuss the "new program" at the College of Medicine with the staff of the state health department. During these meetings the staff were free to ask any questions they wished concerning new developments in medical education in general, or with particular reference to the Department of Preventive Medicine, or the relationship of a medical school to the state health department under such a development. In these discussions, it was important to allay fears that there would be usurpation of health department responsibility.

Anyone who proposes to extend the activity of any organization beyond traditional areas, even for the general good of the public and with legal sanctions, must accept the fact that some individuals, and some organizations will be suspicious of motivation. An earnest attempt to understand the position of the group whose eminence of domain seems to be threatened is a *sine qua non* to the successful accomplishment of a consulting program. That a department of preventive medicine has on its staff personnel who have traditionally been associated only with state health departments is in itself a basis for legitimate concern. In a small state such as Vermont, one can readily understand how a stroke of economic significance might, in its master plan, accommodate the functions of a state health department within the operation of the state medical school. Such fears are well understood, particularly since in a small state it might well make a good deal of sense to avoid duplication and conflict of purpose by just such a consolidation of effort. Needless to say, it takes considerable time, frequent communication, and the use of every opportunity to demonstrate that there is in fact no threat to either personal or professional security. Candid sharing of ideas, opinions, and plans, and explicit rejection of fields of activity that would depart from consultation into service per se, are most disarming when one is faced with serious opposition from groups that must be part and parcel of any endeavor such as this.

In efforts to establish important working relationships in the development of a consultation service, care must be taken to avoid any step that seems to contradict one's announced intention not to usurp the prerogatives of others. One should not, for example, consult with the members of the health commission in a state in which the commissioner of health is responsible to such a commission. However, since in the development of a regional consultation program, suitable legislation might eventually be needed in order to accomplish desired purposes, one might well discuss philosophy and planning with members of the state legislature, and not necessarily only with those who are members of the Public Health Committee of the state legislature. This establishes a frame of reference in the minds of those legislators who, at some future date, may well be important in legislative development. In Vermont, I spent some time with a state senator who was then chairman of the Legislative Committee on Interstate Activity. He and several other senators listened with interest to a description of the developing program at the university and gave it their endorsement. Subsequently, their interest assured progressive development of the interstate program, as well as support of the legislation for the establishment of the Regional Medical Needs Board. Members of the Public Health Committee of the State Legislature were familiar with early developments. Their interest was invaluable in interpretation of the tri-state endeavor on the part of the University of Vermont. It further provided a framework in which the role of a new department of preventive medicine could be defined. Slowly but surely it became understood that the new program at the University of Vermont was limited to consultation. As long as the service element consists of consultation, and the emphasis even within it is placed on research geared toward better teaching, the college of medicine in a state university can fulfill its proper role with the support of all the groups concerned.

Because of the important relationship of the United States Public Health Service to every state health department, the developing program at the University of Vermont was discussed with the New England Director of the United States Public Health Service in the presence of the Vermont Commissioner of Health. The discussion centered largely on interstate cooperation in health matters, its starting point being emphasis on interstate cooperation in rehabilitation—a field which, unfortunately, was not the direct concern of either the United States Public Health Service or the state health department. Discussion of the importance of participation by the *three* health departments in a tri-state program placed a single health department in relation to others. The medical school in one state could not, after all, have plans to absorb the responsibilities and prerogatives of three state health departments.

As progress was slowly made, and as improvement in working relationships continued, it became clear that there would be no necessity to invoke the legal instrument provided by the General Assembly of the State of Vermont. It has gradually become of less and less significance in attempts to meet not only the obligations of the medical school to the state, but to cement relationships which will ultimately produce meaningful and cooperative endeavors in the promotion of health and prevention of disease. From a position of reserved endorsement of the program, the State Department of Health moved toward a more supportive role.

The sequence of events in the strategic development of a consultation program in medical needs emphasizes (1) that legislative sanction, in itself, does not remove barriers to the development of desirable working relationships with other public agencies, and (2) that there must be a willingness to understand the rightful concern of any group over a development which has implications that could reasonably pose a threat to professional and organizational security.

A program arising in one state organization that involves other state organizations, or organizations of other states, does not raise questions of state sovereignty that might be a problem, if a private institution attempted to develop a comparable program.

The people of the states soon begin to feel the influence of the joint effort of state organizations. A state health department may recognize that, while statistics of morbidity and mortality are interesting, the applied influence of the college of medicine in each town and hamlet of the state creates a genuine public desire for more active participation in the fulfillment of needs through the publicly proclaimed cooperation between the state health department and the state medical school. This desire reaches back to the chambers of the legislature. Ultimately, the general public awakens to the fact that efforts to build a healthy state are the best investment their money can make. They begin to see the value of federal participation in programs that cannot be financed by the state alone when it is given in such a way that the sovereignty of the state is maintained, and the moral fiber of individuals or the state is not undermined.

Many such programs could be more realistically and effectively conceived through interstate cooperation. A health department has a major obligation to exercise initiative and resourcefulness if it is to do more than merely keep a routine "police watch" over enforcement of existing regulations or sustain programs which originate with federal legislation. A state health department cooperating with a state university in a regional consultation program has at its disposal, if it cares to use it, an agency which, while an official agency, can serve as "the man without a vested interest."

While the university rendering a consultation service recognizes the importance of abstaining from activity in services areas, it is difficult to maintain a sharp line of demarkation at all times. The problem is rather like that of the teaching hospital when it attempts to separate service costs from costs of research or teaching.

In the development of facilities to increase the availability of day-to-day medical care in rural areas, there is relatively little opportunity for joint participation with the state health department. At the organization meeting of the Regional Medical Needs Committee, it was decided that matters pertaining to the need for day-to-day medical care should be dealt with by the university as a consulting agency and the medical society. For the most part, communities that need greater availability of physicians' services do not have an immediate interest in the full-scale development of general health services in which the participation of the state health department would be essential. At the suggestion of the Vermont Commissioner of Health, joint participation was attempted in the informal organization of the Vermont Council on Physician Placement consisting of the chairman of the Vermont Medical Society's Rural Health Committee, the executive secretary of the Vermont State Medical Society, the Commissioner of

Health or his designee, and myself. It proved to be difficult, however, to get the entire group together at one time for meetings with citizens' committee of a community searching for a physician. More important was the fact that several communities clearly demonstrated that they were not interested in public health services as such but wanted "a doctor when we are sick." After a number of these communities rejected the idea of developing a health center that would include preventive and public health services as well as clinical services, the Vermont Council on Physician Placement ceased to function as such.

In one important area, however, the state health department could participate in efforts to increase the availability of total medical services to a rural area. Once a health center for physicians' services has been established and the community has met its immediate need, the citizens interested and responsible for the health center are much more attuned to consider seriously the values that can accrue from an extension of the scope of services and functions of the center. Timing makes the difference whether or not public health services available from a state health department will be accepted in a community seeking medical care. Unfortunately, few efforts have been made to realize the full potential of the center for the delivery of public health services running the gamut from health education to the organization of community public health clinics. In some instances, a public health nurse visited a health center periodically to discuss matters of mutual interest with the physicians, and school health examination programs and immunization clinics have been moved to the community health center. The clinics, however, are more a function of the professional practice of the physicians than of the development of coordinated public health programs in conjunction with the clinical facilities of the health center.

Occasionally a university consultation program receives requests for advice on medical needs that are of direct concern to a state health department, but which originate from another source. Because the Department of Preventive Medicine had made a study of tuberculosis control for Cumberland County, Maine, which included a general evaluation of tuberculosis control in the state of Maine, the Vermont Tuberculosis and Health Association requested that the Department of Preventive Medicine conduct a similar study in the state of Vermont. Because of the importance of maintaining comfortable working relationships with a local state health department, an appropriate administrative procedure had to be established before the invitation could be accepted.

The president and the executive director of the Vermont Tuberculosis and Health Association were asked to invite representatives from interested organizations to meet at the state health department to discuss this proposal. At the meeting representatives of the state health department, the Vermont Tuberculosis and Health Association, the Vermont State Medical Society, the Department of Social Welfare, and the Department of Institutions were present. The president of the Vermont Tuberculosis and Health Association presided. Following a description of the service rendered to the Cumberland County Tuberculosis and Health Association in Maine, each organization represented stated that a study of the tuberculosis control problem in Vermont would be of great interest, and requested that the Department of Preventive Medicine proceed with such a study.

With each participating group accepting the study and pledging their cooperation in it as needed, the Department of Preventive Medicine proposed that it submit a prospectus. Within three weeks a second meeting was held with the same group, and the prospectus was accepted after minimal modification. At this meeting the Commissioner of Health requested written progress reports on the status of the study. Although this was not practicable because of the lapse of time between the distribution and the return of a sizable number of questionnaires, the Department of Preventive Medicine suggested that each organization appoint one, and no more than one, representative to a committee for continuity of communication. The committee would be summoned when the Department of Preventive Medicine had a significant report to make on the progress of the study, or a report on any particular development that might be of special interest to the group, or to discuss the need for any departure of major consequence from the prospectus as submitted and approved.

The following regulation was passed at a Health Commission meeting on March 21, 1957, a short time before the beginning of the tuberculosis control study.

(1) Except as here-in-after otherwise provided, all information
as to personal facts and circumstances obtained in connection with

the administration of the Vermont State Health Department shall be held confidential and be considered privileged communications, and shall not be divulged or disclosed in any manner what-so-ever without the consent of the individual concerned.

(2) This regulation shall not be construed to prohibit (a) the disclosure of such confidential information in summary, statistical or other form which does not identify particular individuals, or (b) the disclosure after consent by the Commissioner of such confidential information to other agencies or individuals, public or private, that are providing to individuals, needed services. Only such information shall be released as is necessary to achieve the specific purposes for which the disclosure is authorized and after the individual or agency receiving such information has agreed to safeguard the confidential nature of the released information.

Notice of this regulation was circulated by the Commissioner of Health in a form letter to all physicians in the state.

The regulation created certain difficulties in obtaining some data which was important to the prosecution of the study. For example, it was most desirable that one of the social workers of the Department of Preventive Medicine interview patients who had left sanatoria care against advice, but because of the recent ruling of the health commission, it was impossible to obtain the names of these patients. This obstacle was overcome through the assistance and cooperation of the Vermont State Medical Society and the two sanatoria, which helped secure names of patients who had been or were under treatment for pulmonary tuberculosis and who had left institutional care against advice.

Most of the public health nurses of the state health department were reluctant to complete a questionnaire pertaining to their experience and opinions with respect to the existing tuberculosis control program. While this deficit could not be entirely made up, it was possible to gather some information from other nurses working in the public health field such as those of Visiting Nurse Association and school nurses.

One of the major recommendations resulting from this tuberculosis control study for Vermont was to close one of the sanatoria. The incidence and prevalence of tuberculosis did not seem to warrant the economic burden to a small state of maintaining two sanatoria. Prior to the submission of the report on tuberculosis control, the governor submitted legislation to the 1959 General Assembly, recommending that one of the sanatoria be closed. The legislation was eventually passed and contained also, in permissive clauses, another recommendation of the report on tuberculosis control, namely that patients with pulmonary tuberculosis be hospitalized in a general hospital on the advice of the attending physician to the Department of Institutions under whose administrative jurisdiction tuberculosis sanatoria are operated. The recommendation that the remaining tuberculosis sanatorium also ultimately be closed was acted upon in the course of time. A further recommendation that responsibility for the operation of this sanatorium be given to the department of health, and possibly included in a division of chronic diseases under the direction of a physician responsible for medical care of tuberculosis as well as for tuberculosis control programs, was implemented.

Responsibility for conducting a study of a program which is the concern and legal obligation of another state agency naturally raises difficult problems. One can understand the possible reluctance of the state agency to accept advice from a neighbor within the same political and geographic boundaries. Nevertheless, the experience with this study sustained the conviction that a university should be in a position to render objective and unbiased conclusions as an academic, research-oriented body unswayed by considerations of political expediency.

A joint resolution passed by the General Assembly of the State of Vermont in 1959 could become the initiating mechanism for beneficial coordinated action. Because this joint resolution reflects the potential effects of a university consultation program, it is presented here.

***NO. R-63—JOINT RESOLUTION RELATING
TO INTERIM COMMISSION ON TUBERCULOSIS—**

(J. R. H. 35)

Whereas, it appears that tuberculosis in Vermont may continue to be a major health problem for some years to come, despite a decrease in the number of new cases and in debts therefrom in recent years, and

Whereas, advances in the treatment of tuberculosis in recent years tend towards the possibility of eradication or minimizing the incidence of this disease, and

*Unanimous report, submitted March 1961.

178

> *Whereas*, both from a stand point of health and of the alleviation of a drain on the economic resources of a state, it appears desirable that Vermont should make a concerted effort to eradicate tuberculosis and to that end should formulate an up-to-date program based upon a study of the problem in the light of new developments, particularly in the fields of information, case findings, and treatment, and
>
> *Whereas*, the Department of Preventive Medicine of the University of Vermont College of Medicine in conjunction with the Vermont Tuberculosis and Health Association completed a study of tuberculosis control in Vermont, which report is dated February, 1959, now therefore be it
>
> *Resolved by the Senate and House of Representatives:*
>
> That the Department of Preventive Medicine of the University of Vermont College of Medicine in cooperation with the Department of Health and the Vermont Tuberculosis Association, be requested to submit to the 1961 legislature findings and recommendations for a program to eradicate tuberculosis in Vermont.
>
> Approved: June 11, 1959.

One can see expressed in this resolution the interest which the legislature took in a study conducted by one department of its state university. One can understand also the administrative problems which such a resolution presents, particularly since a state department of health could well feel that it is the logical organization to be primarily responsible for such a charge by the legislature. However, after having received the information that the General Assembly had passed such a resolution, and after having discussed the responsibilities contained therein with a representative of the State Health Department and the Vermont Tuberculosis and Health Association, the Department of Preventive Medicine of the state university clearly had to accept the responsibility by appropriate notification to the Speaker of the House and President of the Senate. While recognizing both the responsibility and the ability of the state health department in these matters, the Department of Preventive Medicine had no alternative but to execute its responsibility to the legislature. After considerable discussion, an arrangement was made under which a joint report was submitted to the 1961 legislature as a cooperative endeavor between those organizations named in the resolution.* It is understood that a minority opinion cannot cloud the issues or recommendations, but any minority opinion would certainly be included in the report.*

*See appendix C

G

The Medical Society,
the University, and the Health Department

There is usually no precedent to guide a university when it assumes responsibilities in the actual life of a community or state beyond its traditional role of educating citizens who use their learning in the life of the community and nation as they see fit. There must, therefore, be cooperative endeavor if the university is to apply its academic assets to the realities of problem solving and future planning.

What do we mean by "cooperative"? Simply stated, to cooperate is to act jointly with others toward a goal in which all concur. There can be no cooperation without concurrence—or at least no effective cooperation. This is so because concurrence means a meeting of the minds, an agreement in opinion. Before there can be joint action to a common end, there must be joint acceptance of common endeavor. So-called cooperation without this agreement is nothing but the clamor of wagging tongues in a sea of inactivity.

Cooperation requires joint action based on a meeting of the minds, and the joint action will be only as meaningful as the unanimity and thought behind it are strong. These in turn can be only as strong as the individuals are objective. True cooperation, then, requires an objectivity unsullied by personal ambition, personality clashes, and individual insecurities. This is sometimes difficult to achieve, since as human beings all of us are conditioned by the basic drives of preservation of self and preservation of status, and the desire constantly to improve that status. The mature person can nevertheless cooperate effectively with others toward an objective. When the true elements of cooperation are present, sharing of activity, delegation of responsibility, and assessment of participation become harmonized into a mosaic of complete joint endeavor that leads to efficient accomplishment. Our armed forces move on to victory because each and every man shares the same overriding objective. There has to be cooperation and coordination. In planning for improved health and welfare of a population, members of health departments, medical societies, and medical schools must equally subordinate their individual ambitions to the major objectives, if advances in what is now a relatively impoverished area of our capitalistic society are to be achieved with optimum efficiency and minimum cost.

And what about coordination? Almost by definition, "coordination" implies equality in rank. One who would "coordinate" is one who places things in proper position relative to each other and to the system of which they form parts. There cannot be true coordination without harmonious combination of agents or functions toward the production of a result.

Coordination also inevitably implies a state of "being ordered." Even the most magnanimous sometimes feel reluctant to function in an ordered situation, fearing some loss of executive freedom in a coordinated state of affairs. A struggle over "who is to do the coordinating" can easily ensue. The triad of agencies that are logically concerned with the state of health of the nation—medical societies, health departments, and medical schools—all have important stakes in the discharge of responsibility. There should be no paralyzing jockeying for the position of leader in their coordinated efforts to reach goals they all share.

Now what about planning? Everything which has been stated with respect to cooperation and coordination is prerequisite to any sound planning. What is a plan? It is first of all a draft or form from which expected results can be deduced. Originating from the latin word *planum*, it denotes a flat surface. Here we have a connotation that implies something which is open to view from all sides. There are, in other words, no ridges, corners or slopes that leave doubt or raise questions. Its purpose is clear; it is exposed to critical judgment in all of its facets. A plan also means a method or scheme of action. Since a scheme carries with it the idea of accomplishment by clever contrivance, many people become suspicious of a plan.

In the important relationships among the health department, the university, and the medical society with a shared goal of resolving social pathology (and social pathology includes organic disease), plans refer only to methods by which desirable objectives can be accomplished. Such planning should be exposed in all of its aspects to critical judgment of the three parties. This is particularly the responsibility of the university, if it is to function as the coordinator of the activities of the three agencies. The several interests of medical education, clinical medicine, and public health must be welded into a composite plan for action.

The division of responsibility is ordinarily easy to understand and to accept. There are, of course, always shaded areas in which responsibility for action is obscure. But settling the division of responsibility is a critical phase of planning, involving recognition of the responsibilities of others. The division of responsibility must recognize the primary function of each agency participating. The total approach in planning goes even further, and takes into account the concepts, the needs, and the demands of the individual, his family, and his community as a whole. Planning cannot revolve around the institutional setting alone.

In discussing the relationships among the health department, the university, and the medical society in community or regional endeavor, it is not possible to provide a blueprint for action that will serve every situation. The variety of different factors that would be operating in different situations precludes the development of one blueprint for action. Nevertheless, what was accomplished at Vermont demonstrated conclusively that faculties of universities can work effectively with both medical societies and health departments toward shared objectives.

Although many challenges remain, the university, the medical society, and the health department, working together, can solve many of the problems of medical education, comprehensive medical service, personnel training, and personnel availability.

H

Relationship to Medical Societies

In a university-based consultation program concerned at least in part with the availability of medical care to rural areas, it was as necessary to establish a suitable working relationship with organized medicine in the three states as with the public health departments. The needed endorsement of the program by organized medicine had to be brought about through contact with the officers of the three medical societies.

Physicians are trained to be penetrating in their questions and observations. They are geared to action in the everyday discharge of their responsibilities and they cannot unreasonably defer decisions or cloud their thoughts with extraneous matters irrelevant to the issue. In the daily discharge of professional obligations, the physician cannot afford long, drawn-out procedures which may ultimately indicate a course of action. Responsibility, by and large, must be met at the moment—at the moment at which the patient needs assistance—and specific action affording relief, if not the preservation of life, taken promptly. The physician, consequently, is not likely to "waste" his time, as it were, in nonspecific and nebulous proposals.

The practicing physician is a member of a professional group whose spokesmen impress upon him the alleged importance of maintaining the status quo. In his allegiance to his professional organization, the individual physician often seems to adopt an attitude and a point of view that are not always representative of his basic nature. In taking a stand on legislation that would effect social changes directed at solving problems in health and welfare, the individual physician is likely to act upon the suggestion and, sometimes the persuasion, of the parent professional organization. Yet, in his own practice this physician would certainly not want any of his patients to shoulder an economic burden, or to suffer the consequences of the technological gap between advancement in medical science and the ability to meet its costs. The individual physician is likely to encourage, both for himself and for his patient, a system of security which enhances the comfort and peace of mind of declining years. Each day in his practice the physician has great concern for the individual and his total welfare.

The objectivity which the physician displays in arriving at a diagnosis by no means always characterizes his approach to problems of a social and economic nature, particularly if these problems are the subject of legislation at either the state or federal level. Certainly, the physician does not consciously espouse a different point of view on a question affecting thousands of people, or the nation at large, than he would where only a given individual is involved. Almost all physicians render a significant amount of service on a charitable basis by adjusting their fees to the patient's ability to pay, and take a great deal of satisfaction in meeting this ancient precept of ethics. But many people prefer to risk their health and to endure illness and discomfort rather than seek charitable care or take advantage of the physician's altruism. The physician who adheres to the good old slogans concerning the preservation of individuality, free choice, and doctor-patient relationship, is simply failing to recognize the changing social and economic demands of the twentieth century.

While the self-sufficiency of the physician as an entrepreneur has been undermined by the march of science, technology, and social organization, the ideology of competition and rugged individualism still remains the uncompromising official creed (Rosen, 1958)[8]. In recent years there has been some indication that the philosophy and attitude of the individual physician concerning the social and economic problems affecting the welfare of the individual and the nation, are becoming more consistent with the objectivity of the clinical practice of medicine. This will be true as the parent organization assumes a more liberal posture with respect to the social and economic problems that are confronting the masses in their search for adequate medical care at all ages without affront to personal dignity or failure to take timely advantage of available medical resources. The American Medical Association's adoption in 1960 of a somewhat more open-minded position on a variety of health plans indicates that there has been some increase in objectivity on all problems, not merely those which pertain to the diagnosis and treatment of disease.

Physicians may go through a lengthy conditioning process which militates against their being as objective about social and economic problems as they are about clinical ones. Every medical student comes to learn that Hippocrates is considered to be "the father of medicine." Frequently, even today, the Hippocratic oath is read to medical students as a part of commencement ceremonies, or students actually pledge themselves under the conditions of the Hippocratic oath. Whether this symbol of the ideals of the medical profession is a casual procedure, or whether it is accompanied by an atmosphere which signifies its seriousness of purpose, medical educators would do well to determine whether or not the Hippocratic oath is still applicable. With the finest regard and deepest respect for this physician and his achievements, the assumption cannot be made that aphorisms that applied before Christ continue to have legitimate implications for the twentieth century.

Hippocrates was undoubtedly a very shrewd man (Selwyn-Brown, 1928: Ibid, p. 242). He learned early that he had to become a fully educated man, if he was to be an effective physician. He spent a great deal of time with the philosopher Democritus, who made a great and lasting impression upon him. The systematic study of philosophy, politics and ethics undoubtedly contributed much to his status as a great physician. Many of the teachings of Hippocrates, which caused him to be considered a model for all ages, undoubtedly have some of their roots in his astute judgments. For example, in the Hippocratic oath, he states: "I will not cut persons labouring under the stone, but will leave this to be done by men who are practitioners of this work." Dr. Savas Nittis suggested that this sentence, literally and gramatically translated, means: "I will not castrate, indeed, not even sufferers from the stone. I will keep apart from engaging in this deed." At the time lithotomy was regarded as an abomination and anyone associated with an attempt to relieve suffering by this method would be considered a "quack."

The problem of the incurable patient was a difficult situation for the physician in ancient Greek times. If the physician undertook the treatment of an incurable case, he would be guilty of influencing his unfortunate patient's hopes with false inducements. Such an action would be severely unethical. Consequently, Hippocrates took a point of view which is quite foreign to modern sentiments, namely: "Medicine is the art whereby sufferers may be entirely freed of their ailments and severe attacks of disease medicated, but which should be refused to those persons who are already overwhelmed by illness, since it is clear that in such cases art can be of no avail." Hippocrates thoroughly understood that the history of every science and art has to be secure in our knowledge before we can obtain an intelligent view of its past, and its potentialities and probabilities for the future.

Just how applicable can the Hippocratic oath be in this era of marvelously sophisticated medical science? Let us examine it.

"I swear by Apollo the physician, and Aesculapius, and Hygeia, and Panacea, and all the Gods and Goddesses, that, according to my ability and judgment, I will keep this Oath and this stipulation—to reckon him who taught me this art equally dear to me as my parents, to share my substance with him, and relieve his necessities if required; to look upon his offspring in the same footing as my own brothers, and to teach them this art, if they shall wish to learn it, without fee or stipulation, and that by precept, lecture, and every other mode of instruction, I will impart a knowledge of the art to my own sons, and those of my teachers, and to disciples bound by a stipulation and oath according to the law of medicine, but to none others. I will follow that system of regimen which, according to my ability and judgment, I consider for the benefit of my patients, and abstain from whatever is deleterious and mischievous. I will give no deadly medicine to anyone if asked, nor suggest any such counsel; and in like manner I will not give to a woman a pessary to produce abortion. With purity and holiness I will pass my life and practice my art. I will not cut persons labouring under the stone, but will leave this to be done by men who are practitioners of this work. Into whatever houses I enter, I will go into them for the benefit of the sick, and will abstain from every voluntary act of mischief and corruption; and, further, from the seduction of females or males, of freemen and slaves. Whatever in connection with my professional practice, or not in connection with it, I see or hear, in the life of men, which ought not to be spoken of abroad, I will not divulge, as reckoning that all such should be kept secret. While I continue to keep this Oath unviolated, may it be granted to me to enjoy life in the practice of the art, respected by all men, in all times! But should I trespass and violate this Oath, may the reverse be my lot!"

Quite obviously, many of Hippocrates' commitments are not seriously taken today, nor should they be. The oath encourages a covetousness of medical education which does not obtain today. It calls for a relationship between physicians which is equivalent to that of consanguinity, which is unrealistic, to say the least.

Further, there is a serious question how much the Hippocratic oath should influence a code of ethics. A code of ethics that functions as a protective device for the members of the profession rather than as a protective device for the recipients of medical care is hardly desirable. Yet the Hippocratic oath establishes a fraternity, in a sense, that is not conducive to the aims and objectives of the medical profession as we know it today—and as it is coming to be known. More and more the medical profession is acknowledging the importance of increasing sophistication on the part of the general public in affairs that are medical. For a long time, our code of ethics prevented a physician from assuming a position of leadership in his community by putting himself forward as a knowledgeable person in the field of health and acting as a spokesman for matters of health. The code of ethics would have labeled such positive action as synonymous with "advertising." Now the principles of medical ethics of the American Medical Association implicitly recognize the importance of the public's awareness of health matters, and further, or making every effort to make available to the public the benefits of professional attainments. It can be assumed that the availability of the benefits of professional attainment is not confined to technical skills, but extends to general health education for the public.

While there is much in the Hippocratic oath for which all good men will strive, this oath should surely now be modified in keeping with the present status of medicine in a world in which it strives to retain a position of paramount confidence and respect. Hippocrates himself modified an earlier oath to meet the needs of his time. Babylonian physicians had used a similar oath, and it appears to historians that it has come down to us from a remote part of the Stone Age. There have been a number of modifications of the Hippocratic oath, such as the Christian Doctors' Oath, the Arabian Doctors' Oath, the Indian form of the oath, and the British Oath (Selwyn-Brown 1928: Ibid, p. 242). Physicians, because of their close association with the powers of birth and death, are considered to be and in fact are, in a way, a special class. But the oath physicians of today and tomorrow take, should not imply secrecy or special bonds beyond those which serve the purpose of sympathetic altruistic service to humanity.

In the early 1500s Paracelsus acknowledged the importance of the relationship of the physician to his colleagues through organization. He exhorted physicians to experiment, to study, and to think for themselves, and to do whatever their own judgment indicated was proper. He deplored the "fetish" of custom and reverence for authority, and branded as imperative a freedom of thought which would also develop a new branch of endeavors.

Medical societies have been in existence as long as there have been physicians. Even the primitive medicine man had his societies. The American Indians developed medical societies to a high degree. The Australians and South Sea Islanders, the Africans, and many other modern savages have them. Only in recent years have medical societies become institutions for the promotion of medical science. For too long they were purely social groups designed primarily to protect the social and economic status of their members.

It was the relationship of the physician to his ideals and to his representative organization that was extremely important in working with the officers of medical societies in the establishment and endorsement of a consultation program.

As a physician myself, I already had some understanding of this relationship, and could, I felt, approach the officers of medical societies on a basis of comprehension and respect. Naturally, I did not expect prompt acclaim for each idea I proposed. Physicians are trained to weigh and examine carefully. One must remember, too, that while medicine is a profession of tremendous social action, it is the individual physician rather than his organization that takes the lead. Putting oneself in the position of the person to be convinced not only fosters greater insight into his point of view, but also helps materially to disarm him.

Organized medicine in the three northern New England states showed remarkable and praiseworthy interest and cooperation in the development of a program that was to explore the possibilities of resolving problems in medical needs on a regional basis. The annual reports of the Vermont State Medical Society reflect the seriousness of purpose with which the physicians cooperated in this endeavor. The medical societies of Maine and New Hampshire were equally cooperative. It is understood that being "cooperative" does not mean immediate acquiescence in every new thought or action proposed. It would indeed be surprising and distressing, if a group of physicians failed to display, through their organized association, some degree of inquisitiveness, interrogation, and investigation. The strongest foundations are built where acceptance of ideas is gained by the reasoned conquest of doubt and disagreement.

In the 1956 Annual Report of the Vermont State Medical Society, the president reports the establishment of the Regional Medical Needs Committee in May of 1955. In the same annual report a page is given to the discussion of the establishment of the Vermont Council on Physician Placement. Also in that report the president mentioned the concern of the Department of Preventive Medicine at the medical school for needed amendment to the Hill-Burton Act, and reported that the council of the medical society endorsed the department's efforts to effect such an amendment. At the same Council meeting, a tri-state (Maine, New Hampshire, and Vermont) placement service was envisioned to be directed by the medical school. This was brought to a motion and passed. The tri-state physician placement service as a formally organized activity would logically follow the study of the medical needs of Maine, New Hampshire, and Vermont. For important reasons of strategy, the formal study of the region as a whole had been deferred, despite the usual public health practice calling first for a careful survey to define problems, the scope of problems, and probable solutions. Once working relationships were well established in the region a formal survey could take place.

In the 1957 Annual Report of the Vermont State Medical Society, the following comments were made by the president: "State legislative matters had the active attention of the Council this past year. It has been most heartening to see the Council willing to enter actively into such matters. The Tri-State Medical Needs Act was enacted with Society support. Maine and New Hampshire cooperatively enacted similar measures. This is a forward step for medical education centered in our U.V.M. College of Medicine." In the same annual report, there is a four-page discussion of the proposal that the Department of Preventive Medicine be responsible for a study of tuberculosis control. Then there follows: "The Vermont Tuberculosis and Health Association has sponsored plans for a thorough survey of the tuberculosis problem in Vermont. The committee representative of the State Medical Society has aided in forming these plans and presenting them to the Council of the State Society. The Council passed the following resolution:

"A motion was made to approve the survey, providing that in addition to the criteria set up for the survey, the conclusions would indicate a proper, future program for the association to pursue."

Prior to the endorsement of legislation to establish the Regional Medical Needs Board, the annual session of the House of Delegates of the Vermont State Medical Society, meeting on October 7, 1956, chose to table this subject when there was some objection to the establishment of the Regional Medical Needs Board. Subsequently, there was full endorsement and support of this legislation, as reported earlier. The Council had appointed a committee of three to act for the Council on this bill, and the bill was passed.

In the 1958 Annual Report of the Vermont State Medical Society, considerable discussion is given to the need for amendment of the Hill-Burton Act in order to allow funds for diagnostic and treatment centers to be utilized at the local rural level. The Council then went on record as approving the intents of an amendment to Public Law 482 which would enable rural areas to receive an equitable share of diagnostic and treatment center funds for the establishment of health centers.

In the same annual report, the Council endorsed the submission of letters to the Governors of Maine, New Hampshire, and Vermont concerning reciprocity of payment for indigent cancer patients in these states.

In the Vermont State Medical Society's annual report for 1959, a progress report is given on the Vermont tuberculosis control study in which it is pointed out that the study had been completed, and was receiving close scrutiny by many interested persons. It was further pointed out that the study was part of the basis of a continuing study requested by the legislature during the next year and one-half.

Thus, it can be seen that the medical societies were actively participating in the regional medical needs program established and operated by the Department of Preventive Medicine.

While the Vermont Council for Physician Placement was short-lived, the way in which this joint approach to requests for help from communities was initiated and attempted for Vermont may prove interesting. In a 1956 memorandum to the Council of the Vermont State Medical Society I pointed out:

"Since the establishment of the Regional Medical Needs Committee in May of 1955, every effort has been made to approach requests from communities so that they appreciate the fact that the medical profession, through its participation, is actively engaged in seeking solutions to rural medical needs. Through the efforts of the executive secretary of the Vermont Medical Society, physicians seeking areas in which to practice medicine and communities seeking physicians have received assistance. Requests for such assistance reach both the medical society and the medical school.

"To provide assistance in a field of mutual endeavor on an organized basis, it is requested that the Council authorize participation in requests for assistance in the following manner:

"1. The executive secretary and a member of the rural health committee to meet with the director of health studies of the medical school [the author] and the commissioner of health or his designated representative(s), to discuss problems of a community requesting assistance. The director of health studies will obtain information about the community for the other members, and arrange for them to meet with interested citizens regarding assistance.

"2. Because of the problem of travel, it is hoped that the Council will authorize the chairman of the rural health committee to appoint a representative when it would be difficult for him or a member of the rural health committee to meet in Burlington, or to visit a community. Such a representative presumably would keep the chairman of the rural health committee informed.

"Experience in Maine and New Hampshire in dealing with rural medical needs indicates that:

"1. Small rural communities can be helped to help themselves when given a little guidance and direction.

"2. The university representative has the time to spend on gathering information and working out details for the community concerned.

"3. The health department will contribute by way of advising, especially with reference to Hill-Burton funds, and lending assistance through personnel such as a health educator.

"4. The coordinated efforts of university, medical society, and health department demonstrate ability to meet medical needs at the local level."

A letter from the executive secretary of the Vermont State Medical Society indicated the Council's approval of the approach to assisting communities needing better availability of day-to-day medical care. As noted previously, however, this council for physician placement did not work satisfactorily.

The attempt to establish a Vermont Council on Physician Placement was not entirely a failure. It did provide a medium through which representatives of a state health department, a medical society, and a medical school could discuss and consider problems of mutual concern. It was an asset in focusing the attention of relevant groups upon the priorities which the general public set in meeting their needs for day-to-day medical care.

Despite the demise of the Vermont Council on Physician Placement, the Department of Preventive Medicine continued to work with the medical societies of the three states on the problems of availability of physicians to communities. The procedure was to consult with the executive secretary or the executive director of the medical society on an inquiry that came to the department for assistance in obtaining a physician. The medical societies are always most cooperative and supportive in efforts to work with communities to obtain physicians. There has been only one instance in which a local practicing physician obviously objected to any competition in the area although there was need for another physician. In this particular instance, the problem was discussed with the physicians in the area, one of whom was the one making the objections. Under the system of free enterprise in the practice of medicine, one physician can make it very difficult for another physician to establish himself in a community even though his services may be needed there. In this case this was particularly true because of the part-time effort of one of the physicians. This could have been a test case in determining the action of a medical society. No formal survey of the area was conducted, however, because the citizens' committee did not pursue the matter. Had a survey been conducted, and had the survey indicated a clear need for additional physicians in the area, it would necessarily have been a matter for the state medical society to advise whether or not procedures should be implemented to obtain another physician. Or, the problem might have been brought before the Regional Medical Needs Board for the establishment of a policy that could apply in other situations where a physician was monopolizing the area in order to safeguard his own level of practice.

When a university is involved in a consultation service, particularly one relating to the availability of medical care, the medical school cannot fail to become interested in the practicing physician's business. In establishing working relationships with the medical society, the medical school's attitude and approach must necessarily be one of understanding and support of the physician's responsibility to his public, and at the same time it must be concerned with the needs of the public for increased availability of adequate medical care. It was undoubtedly this kind of dual loyalty that gave rise to an early impression that the medical school might be attempting to engage in the corporate practice of medicine. This attitude was undoubtedly reinforced by the school's recommendations that communities build facilities in order to attract physicians. Slowly this misconception was overcome. To do so required understanding not only of the individual physician, but also of organized medicine at the county level, the state level, and the national level. There is no measurement of the degree to which the prestige of physicians, as reflected in popular magazines, has been lowered because of the negativism of the parent organization. One can speculate how much this negativism has to do with general public dissatisfaction with the delivery of medical care. The American Medical Association unfortunately has not always been mindful of the increasing sophistication of the general public in its concern for the rewards of total and comprehensive medical care.

In 1922 the American Medical Association officially disapproved the maternity and infancy (Sheppard-Towner) act, which was designed to improve the nutrition of children and mothers during the childbearing period. In 1927, the Committee on Costs of Medical Care (Rosen, 1958)[11] split into a majority and a minority when it made its recommendations. The majority favored medical and hospital care insurance on a voluntary basis until adequate experience could be accumulated to serve as a sound basis for a comprehensive system based on compulsory tax deductions. The majority also approved group medical practice organized around health centers. It favored government grants-in-aid to provide hospitals, doctors, and nurses in poor and thinly populated areas. It recommended that the cost of medical care for the indigent, the tuberculous, and the mentally ill be borne by the state. While the minority agreed in many respects with the majority, it had little to offer that was constructive. It reaffirmed the opposition of the medical and dental organizations to prepaid medical care even on a voluntary basis, and objected particularly to the proposal for group practice. The minority opposed insurance plans unless sponsored and controlled by organized medicine. The *Journal of the American Medical Association* went even further and indicted the majority report as "inciting to revolution." In 1935, however, the House of Delegates of the American Medical Association encouraged local medical organizations to establish plans for the provision of adequate medical service to all the people, adjusted to present economic conditions, by voluntary budgeting to meet the cost of illness. . . . Thus, it seems to have been the pattern that the American Medical Association has followed, not led, and has moved forward only when pressure has been brought to bear for something to be done. This is not the position a professional organization should be in. It is a known and understood fact that one cannot usually legislate a moral or social code, but that legislation will follow in the wake of demand. A professional organization should not follow through under duress, but rather should take the lead in pressing for the establishment of ways and means to accomplish the purposes for which it supposedly exists. When a professional organization reaches a state when it can be indicted by the United States Department of Justice for restraint of lawful practice and conspiracy to prevent independent endeavor to meet problems of health needs of the nation, then something is very wrong. One might expect such an indictment, which was lodged in 1938 and later upheld by the United States Supreme Court, to be brought against a trade or business corporation but not against a professionally oriented service agency. Recent trends indicate that the fountainhead of American medicine is unlikely to find itself again in such an embarrassing position. It is hopeful that these trends will lead to open negotiation, discussion, and pursuit of solutions to problems of national concern (Goldmann, 1945)[12].

Because of its interest in regional medical needs, the department had to work closely with the American Medical Association. The philosophy and natural bent of the individual physician to serve mankind were in great evidence. But the influence of the body corporate and body politic all too often was thrown behind an interference that would, if it could, prevent amendment to national legislation to make it possible for rural areas to have equitable consideration in the expenditure of federal funds for diagnostic and treatment centers which they, as well as urban citizens, had contributed.

While on the national level the American Medical Association has opposed needed legislation, this has not been the stand of local medical societies. The medical societies of Maine, New Hampshire, and Vermont did promote and, as a matter of fact, introduced legislation to establish the quasi-official Regional Medical Needs Board. Furthermore, these three medical societies, individually and through joint action on the Regional Medical Needs Board, endorsed efforts to amend Public Law 482, Title VI of the United States Public Health Service Act, to enable rural areas that did not need hospitals but rather facilities that would provide ambulatory, day-to-day medical care to secure funds for diagnostic and treatment centers. It can be seen, again and again, that the individual physician and often the local state medical society as well, behave, think, and act quite differently from the national parent. The Maine Medical Association, particularly through the efforts of its executive director, Dr. Daniel F. Hanley, assisted a great deal toward the suitable amendment of Public Law 482, pertaining to diagnostic and treatment center provision for rural areas. The northern New England medical societies demonstrated an awareness of the importance of the role of the physician in political life by taking the lead in developing and proposing legislation. No longer can the individual physicians in the solo practice of medicine (a feature of "the good old days") be the instrumental, by themselves, for meeting the health needs of a nation.

There is much that still needs to be done by joint effort for appropriate legislation. Medical practice acts in many states are antiquated and should be updated. Adjoining states should have compacts of medical practice licensure. Legislation is needed to meet the problems of medical economics. There is a need for legislation to improve the status of management of long-term illness. None of these needs can be met simply by the good will of the individual physician.

Efforts to meet medical needs through physician placement should be integrated. One model is the program developed at the University of Vermont. There are others. Problems in physician placement, physician education, community education regarding medical practice and medical needs are all efforts which can, and should, command concerted action by organized medicine to bring about position enabling legislation. It is possible to establish acceptable social legislation that is not subject to the stigma of "socialized medicine."

In this connection there is a very valuable service which could be organized for the benefit of medical societies through the joint efforts of the university and the health department. In these days of rapid development of social legislation, physicians who are asked to endorse such legislation often have not had the time to study the full implications of legislation either at the state level or at the federal level. State medical societies frequently ask or encourage their members to write or to send telegrams to their congressmen supporting the position of the parent organization. All too often, the individual physician goes along without having read the entire bill or having had the opportunity to hear an objective analysis of the pros and cons of the proposed legislation.

It would assist the physician considerably if state and county medical societies had available to them a lecture service that could present at their meetings an objective, unbiased analysis of legislation important to the individual physician. The state health department could provide such a service. The state health department is accustomed to working with state and federal legislation and to interpreting such legislation for its own guidance and action as required under law. The university through its law school or department of political science could also cooperate in presenting an objective analysis of pending legislation. Such a program would result in clearer comprehension of the implications behind social legislation. Thus the individual physician, who is wholly preoccupied with the discharge of his professional responsibilities, would be in a better position to evaluate. The present tendency to adopt a position without individual objective analysis of all of the factors involved is the very antithesis of the physician's usual approach to problems in his professional field. Medicolegal forums for the discussion and objective analysis of important pending social legislation would be a very effective postgraduate experience, and one which most physicians would accept and thoroughly appreciate. At the same time, these forums would bring to the practicing physician the sort of effort now being made in medical schools to give some time, though not nearly enough, to the analysis of important social legislation in the teaching of medical care systems and programs.

In the instance of a regional medical needs program in northern New England, the practicing doctors' business has become the medical school's interest. In rural areas, of course, this must revolve around the general practice of medicine since the population is generally too small to support division of labor and specialization in practice. The interest of necessity encompasses an indirect approach to the problem of medical economics, particularly in rural areas. For, wherever there are, at each local level, adequate services on an ambulatory basis, including the essence of preventive medicine through health promotion, early diagnosis, and prompt treatment, there is a beneficial result in terms of long-range reduction of cost.

In a number of areas the coordinated efforts of the university and health department and the medical society could help to solve current problems. The Rural Health Committee of the Vermont State Medical Society has, in the course of its meetings, cited a number situations which need attention. These include health education, understanding of the physician's responsibility and his needs in order to do a better job, environmental sanitation, nutrition, dental service, adequate medical service, first aid and home nursing, availability of health officers who are trained and equipped for this task, care of the aged, and farm safety. These are but a few of the areas in which there can be increased cooperative and integrated activity on the part of the medical society, the health department, and the university.

There are many ways in which the university, as a consulting agency, can establish field research to assist in the analysis and solution of problems pertaining to the adequacy of medical care. It has already been pointed out that a formal survey of the region in order to obtain an analysis of current inadequacies, with recommendations for long-range planning on those problems which cannot be solved immediately, had not been carried out. It was important that this study include review of the mobility of physicians from one type of practice to another, an evaluation of medical care in communities of comparable and varying sizes with particular emphasis upon the concepts of the lay public and their medical needs, the manner in which they are currently met, and opinions concerning ways in which they might be better met.

The development of pleasant working relationships with the county and state medical societies was an encouraging indication that problems of health and welfare can also be dealt with nationally, if organized medicine is approached with understanding of the individual physician in his capacity as a clinician. Frank appraisal of hurdles and obstacles leaves one with the conviction that they have been greatly exaggerated. One finds that one can work successfully with these men and women of great humanitarian concern whose combined efforts can lead to action of great significance. Much necessary and desirable action cannot take place without their active participation—and fortunately, this participation, while rightfully critical at first, is ultimately given for the successful execution of a health and welfare program.

Conclusion

All activity in an academic institution is without logical basis unless it ultimately serves the primary purposes of teaching and research. Because of its primary function of teaching and research the university in turn has an institutional responsibility to the public. This was the premise on which a formally organized program in consultation to a region in problems of medical needs was initially established.

A faculty that is involved in the cold, hard business of applying its skills to practical situations is not likely to become sterile in its approach to teaching. This is the constant argument of clinicians who regard an opportunity for continuing clinical practice as a *sine qua non* of effective teaching. While definite, committed full-time teaching without private clinical practice does not preclude effective teaching, such orientation to adequate performance does present a substantive argument for the combination of academic and clinical medicine. When medical training becomes truly university centered, the full-time, clinical academician encounters sufficient exposure to clinical medicine in the discharge of well-organized supervisory activity.

The true academic life is characterized by a leisurely approach to problems and solutions. A full-time faculty participating in a consultation program should have the time not only to think through problems encountered in consultation, but also to think about and to execute effective research. An active consultation program provides many situations out of which there can develop research that is pertinent to both immediate and long-range solutions to problems.

The value of a consultation program to students is directly proportional to the degree with which ideas, concepts and problems are presented from experience. In the presentation of subject matter which is readily recognized by the student as "clinical," there is likely to be utilization of material from the faculty member's personal experience in providing medical care or in consultation. Likewise, there should be active and "live" amphitheater presentation of material which may be several steps removed from the student's concept of clinical medicine, but which nevertheless is an extremely important factor in teaching medicine.

The consultation program of a university then is a "field laboratory." Otherwise, there is no real basis for a university to develop a consultation program. While the present instance deals with an administratively organized program within a medical school, there is no reason to exclude possibilities for comparable consultation programs in other fields of endeavor.

Major activity in such a consultation program denotes implications for change in medical school curricula. There can be no real understanding of medical education's needs to meet demands and needs of the future, unless there is an understanding of the arena in which the many graduates of medical schools ultimately face the conflict of holding fast to ideals of medical practice and the realities of problems and pressures in medical practice, the foremost of which are in the area of medical economics, long-term illness and gerontology.

Consultation in Health Needs of a Region; Practice, Problems, and Pressures

That there was established a consultation program in medical needs, extending through the states of Maine, New Hampshire and Vermont, is a certainty. As a matter of fact, the demands from the region reached the point where not all requests could be met. The acceptance of such a program was amply demonstrated. The position then was one of moving to a careful study of the region as a whole, the objective being to define total needs with stated proposals as to ways and means in which this northeastern area could enhance public health and medical care activity through even closer, formalized interstate relationships. Such an evaluation necessarily has to follow acceptance on the part of official and voluntary groups. That such activity on the part of the medical school was acceptable was certainly without question.

This does not mean that careful vigilance must not be maintained with regard to differentiation of consultation and service. It does not mean either that all activities in which an academic group might become engaged, both for benefits that accrue to intramural, academic activity and to the region as a whole, are not going to be carefully scrutinized by individuals and organizations concerned. Human nature never gives carte blanche to activities that could eventuate an alteration of organizational patterns. This concern has been much in evidence throughout the establishment of a department of preventive medicine with a regional consultation program. Success in the establishment of the department with extension activity was testimony to the cooperation and intellectual curiosity of members of medical societies and state departments of health.

In any consultation program, there are certain to be problems and pressures which oftentimes stem from fears and fantasy on the part of individuals and organizations. The true mark of the university must extend into the community area of consultation, and do all within its power to influence favorably actions for the best long-range results. This must be the case even at the expense of loss of momentary "popularity." Compromises are in order but only when they do not affect adversely a desirable end result.

There was established a consultation program in medical needs at the University of Vermont, originating with the Department of Preventive Medicine. It was a program based on skills to be provided by a department of preventive medicine with an interest in medical care problems.

There developed a continuing quasilegal organization, the Regional Medical Needs Board. Through its organization, there should be continuing contact between medical society, health department, and medical schools.

The system that was developed is important in its reliance upon skills and organization rather than upon a given individual.

A plan of organization which emphasizes the system, rather than the individual, is likely to meet with success. Even the most magnanimous are not likely to be without envy and prejudice, if a program is egocentric in nature; that is, seeming to "building" an individual rather than a department or a program. There is always the necessity of taking whatever steps seem indicated to avoid impressions of personal aggrandizement.

There remains in the consultation program, or as a result of it, the important matter of a formal study of the region with proposals for interstate endeavor. There is the important necessity of attempting to establish a tri-state physician placement organization as the pooled effort of the three medical societies. It is reasonable that the principal place of business of such an organization should be at the four-year medical school in Vermont. The problems in physician placement were well understood by the department at the university. This department could continue its interests or it could pass them on to another organization with intermittent consultation service as required. Once patterns have been established through such a consultation program, it is important that the university relinquish, whenever indicated, a program which has been developed through study. Such may well be the case with the physician placement service in the interest of an academic department reaching into other areas of endeavor which could in turn be adopted and carried on by other groups.

The matter of legislation, particularly as it pertains to Public Law 482, should still be pursued. The amendment of Public Law 482 in order to bring diagnostic and treatment center facilities into rural areas is important. A formal study of rehabilitation potential in a tri-state cooperative endeavor should be pursued. These are skills and overwhelming assets at the Crotched Mountain Foundation in Greenfield, New Hampshire, which should be taken into serious consideration in the development of rehabilitation programs in Maine, New Hampshire, and Vermont.

These were the immediate interests stemming from the development of a consultation program in a department of preventive medicine. There are certain to be many other endeavors of potential interest. The important factors are that a base was established and adequate, working relationships developed to provide the climate for remaining alert to potential activity, not only in one state through its university, but to a natural region as a result of the activities of a department of preventive medicine.

It is not the purpose of this book to deal specifically with the growing gap between technological development in medicine and the economic and social advances that would bring the benefits of that development within the reach of every member of our population. That gap can, and undoubtedly will be bridged without loss of moral or professional strength by either individuals or special population groups.

Among the real barriers to the availability of medical care, in addition to economic factors, are such social factors as the attitudes of both physicians and patients. These compound the problem of the skewed distribution of physicians. They further complicate the deficiencies in interstate cooperative and endeavor which could be overcome by cooperative thought, planning, and action so that we could realize the potential that is within our reach were it not for such human frailties as self-interest and the desire to preserve individual status or group identification without appropriate regard for the inherent obligation of the individual or the group.

In considering the health needs of a region to which it seeks to extend consulting services, a university should not be bound by traditional concepts of medical attention—which incidentally give only episodic care to given groups within the population. The facts that children up to a certain age may receive fairly regular health maintenance; and that women in certain years of their lives, notably the reproductive years, may receive episodic attention to health maintenance; and that industrial workers may receive varying degrees of regular health maintenance, do not mean that there are no longer large numbers of people who need adequate attention. This country, like many of the so-called underdeveloped nations, has major problems at both extremes of the life cycle—children and aged persons. There is no one group in the population, particularly in rural areas, that is not in need of coordinated forces that will function in such a way as to bring adequate, daily delivery of medical care and regular attention to health maintenance.

While there are realistic barriers to medical care, and to efficient and adequate health maintenance in rural areas, and to some extent in sections of urban areas, there are some barriers that are only those of fantasy. Many attitudes toward so-called socialized concepts of medical care serve as barriers to the people's rights to a healthful life and the pursuit of happiness. There has been no profession of greater social action than the medical profession; this is shown in the lengthened life of our people. It is, however, through the medical profession's very social action of preserving and prolonging life, which must continue through intensive biological and social science research, that the barrier to responsibility for types of medical care other than resolution of pathology alone must be removed. Too many physicians in their student days, and in their postgraduate years, have acquired a zeal for this one important, but nevertheless narrow, approach to the discharge of the physician's responsibility. It is their strictly pathological orientation which has fostered misunderstanding of the fact that a physician's responsibility encompasses maintenance of health as well as resolution of pathology.

Health needs, in contradistinction to so-called medical needs, must be borne in mind when a university-based consultation service is established. This inevitably means that the consultation program will be concerned with voluntary and public or official groups of the region, which already have obligations for the promotion of health and assistance with availability of physicians and medical care services. This brings the university establishing such a service in touch with the small voluntary "citizens-for-action" groups, rural farm organizations, the local part-time health officer, the district health office of the state department of health, and the county and state medical societies. If there is a searching approach to ways in which a program of consultation may be of assistance to a small rural community, or on an interstate basis to states, the national organizations of both public and voluntary organized groups soon enter the picture. This must of necessity be so, if the responsibility assumed in consulting at the local level is to be executed in such a way as to reveal and deal with basic problems in lack of adequate health and medical services. Health needs must of necessity be taken into serious account, along with the less encompassing term, medical needs.

Hospital facilities, even in rural areas, are not lacking, partly because of the construction undertaken under the Hill-Burton legislation. Indeed, it might be said that there is an overabundance of these facilities. One could say that in many, perhaps most, areas there is no further need for hospital construction. It is another matter to consider facilities on a regional basis which would assure early diagnosis and prompt treatment, along with health promotion, for population groups that neither need, nor could support, financially or professionally, a general hospital. Heavy expenditure in bricks and mortar is not required; rather, genuine cooperative endeavor for the promotion of health among the sparsely populated areas is needed.

Rural areas need adequate midway stations between the home and the hospital. There is a need for a mechanism that will bring the physician into small town areas to care for a public that can and should remain ambulatory in its medical care without the necessity of greater expenditure on the costly overhead of the hospital. There are facilities that can meet this problem, developed and organized on the principle of the nonprofit, charitable, voluntary hospital organization.

The solution to problems of need and demand is clear to those who hold a literal and unselfish interpretation of professional service for the health and welfare of each individual, regardless of where he may choose to live and work. Needs to be met complicate the problems because the solutions often cannot be found within the framework of existing traditional approaches. Availability of personnel with modified technical training to meet specific needs demands compromise, but compromise without mediocrity. Just as the dental hygienist has assumed an appreciable degree of responsibility that was at one time wholly that of the dentist; just as the nurse's aide and the licensed practical nurse have assumed much of the responsibility that was once wholly that of the graduate and registered professional nurse, so there are areas which may have at their disposal the services of certified personnel technically trained to an extent that would meet the requirements of health needs. Both current organizational structure and types of personnel create complex problems in meeting regional medical needs, and they will continue to do so as long as unrealistic criteria are applied regardless of where services are delivered. The requirements for sound practice are not the same at all levels. The general physician's office, for example, does not need the services of a registered laboratory technician. Yet, there are those who insist that a "laboratory technician" be used even when a "laboratory aide" could satisfactorily perform all the laboratory procedures needed on a routine basis.

These complex problems are not relieved by the attitudes now current in the medical profession both with respect to their specific professional responsibilities and to developments they carelessly consider "socialized," and presumably evil. If meaningful solutions are to be found, physicians will have to think as objectively about social and economic problems as they now do about specific organic illness. The general public may not necessarily understand why physicians cling to these attitudes, but its nostalgia for the days of the "good old family physician" certainly expresses its dissatisfaction. As individuals, many physicians are socially conscious of their obligation and responsibility to a society to which changing medical practice must necessarily be adapted. The dicta of the organization of a major professional group often do not represent the attitudes of individual physicians. On the one hand, there is great public expectation of what the physician can accomplish technically as a result of the tremendous scientific strides that have been made. On the other hand, the public also wants personal interest and concern from the physician. This existed in the days when lack of technology per force brought the physician in to a much closer personal relationship to his patient. The demand on the part of the public now is to have the technical services that are available at a cost which it can afford without loss of personal relationship between physician and patient.

The development of every field, including public health and clinical medicine, has been enriched by the thoughts and deeds of men who projected, almost prophetically, the needs of the years beyond their time. Each succeeding generation has only to build upon the accomplishments of the past, and to bring to fruition through appropriate implementation the ideas and ideals of men and women whose period of influence extends beyond their three score years and ten. Cicero asked: "What were the life of man did we not combine present events with their predecessors in past time?" When we pause in the midst of the busy preoccupations of our daily living to think, we realize that a social life of little more than 30,000 years is a brief span in comparison with two and one-quarter billion years of geological time. It would be remarkable indeed if we did not feel that there is much still to be accomplished before we can hope to be within reach of an ordered state of affairs that would meet the needs of mankind in a manner that is neither weakening to the spirit nor debilitating to the social fiber. The important thing is that each generation maintain a purposeful expenditure of time, thought and energy in order to avoid drifting onto undesirable shoals. Each generation has had, and will continue to have, leaders whose bold foresight charts navigable streams of civilization. Purposeful expenditure of time and energy precludes the distortion of goals, and the methods by which they shall be attained, by personal fear, anxiety, or prejudice. Human frailties will always be with us. Appropriate social action and legislation can meet the demands of a changing demography and economy without deterioration of the social order as a whole.

Appendix A

Community Medicine: Organization and Application of Principles

SUBCHAPTER 1. MEDICAL NEEDS COMPACT

SECTION

701. Purpose—Article I.
702. Tri-state regional medical needs board—Article II.
703. When operative—Article III.
704. Officers; duties; powers; conduct of business—Article IV.
705. Data; reports; research; fees—Article V.
706. Gifts—Article VI.
707. Separability of provisions—Article VII.
708. Duration; withdrawal of membership—Article VIII.
709. Default—Article IX.

SUBCHAPTER 2. PROVISIONS RELATING TO COMPACT

741. Ratification.
742. Copies.
743. Exchange and filing of documents.
744. Report.

§ 701. Purpose—Article I

In order to provide advisory service to voluntary and official health agencies and educational institutions concerned with health, relating to policies concerned with the promotion, preservation and restoration of health and to insure the availability of day-to-day medical care where there is need in the rural areas of the compacting states.

HISTORY

Source. 1957, No. 154, § 1.

§ 702. Tri-state regional medical needs board—Article II

There is hereby created and established a Tri-State Regional Medical Needs Board which shall be the agency of each state party to the compact. The board shall be a body corporate and politic having the powers, duties and jurisdiction herein enumerated and such other and additional powers as shall be conferred upon it by the concurrent act or acts of the compacting states. The board shall consist of the president, vice-president and president-elect of the medical societies of Vermont and New Hampshire and the president, president-elect and executive director of the Maine Medical Association; the commissioners of health of the three states; the deans of the University of Vermont and Dartmouth Medical Schools; the chairman of the curriculum committee and director of health studies of the University of Vermont College of Medicine, the latter two without vote.

HISTORY

Source. 1957, No. 154, § 1.

Cross references. Agencies attached to governor's office, see § 1a of Title 3.

§ 703. When operative—Article III

This compact shall become operative immediately at such time as the last of the three compacting states shall have executed it in the form which is in accordance with the laws of the respective compacting states.

HISTORY

Source. 1957, No. 154, § 1.

Cross references. Ratification of compact, see § 741 of this title.

§ 704. Officers; duties; powers; conduct of business—Article IV

The board shall annually elect from its members a chairman,

and vice-chairman, and shall appoint and at its pleasure remove
or discharge said officers. It may appoint and employ an executive
secretary and may employ such stenographic, clerical, technical
or legal personnel as shall be necessary, and at its pleasure may
remove or discharge such personnel. It shall adopt a seal and
suitable by-laws and shall promulgate any and all rules and regulations which may be necessary for the conduct of its business. It
may maintain an office or offices within the territory of the compacting states and may meet at any time or place. Meetings shall
be held at least once in each calendar year. A majority of the
members shall constitute a quorum for the transaction of business
but no action of the board imposing any obligation on any compacting state shall be binding unless a majority of the members
from such compacting state, shall have voted in favor thereof.
Where meetings are planned to discuss matters relevant to problems of rural medical needs of only certain of the compacting
states, the board may vote to authorize special meetings of the
board members of such states. The board shall keep an accurate
account of all receipts and disbursements and shall make an annual report to the governor and the legislature of each compacting state, setting forth in detail the operations and transactions
conducted by it pursuant to this compact and shall make recommendations for any legislative action deemed by it advisable, including amendments to the statutes of the compacting states
which may be necessary to carry out the intent and purposes of
this compact. The board shall not pledge the credit of any compacting state without the consent of the legislature thereof given
pursuant to the constitutional process of said state. The board
may meet any of its obligations in whole or in part with funds
available to it under Article VI of this compact; provided, that the
board takes specific action setting aside such funds prior to the
incurring of any obligation to be met in whole or in part in this
manner. Except where the board makes use of funds available to
it under Article VI hereof, the board shall not incur any obligations for salaries, office, administrative, traveling or other expenses prior to the allotment of funds by the compacting states
adequate to meet the same. Each compacting state reserves the
right to provide hereafter by law for the examination and audit of
accounts of the board. The board shall appoint a treasurer who
may be a member of the board, and disbursements by the board
shall be valid only when authorized by the board and when vouch-

ers therefor have been signed by the executive secretary and countersigned by the treasurer. The executive secretary shall be custodian of the records of the board with authority to attest to and certify such records or copies thereof.

The board shall study and consider for implementation and operation on a tri-state cooperative basis program to promote, preserve and restore health in the rural areas of the compacting states. Any program deemed advisable for implementation and operation on a tri-state basis shall be submitted to each of the three legislatures with the endorsement of the members of the board and such program shall include therein an analysis of administrative and operational costs and a proposed division of costs on an equitable basis for each of the three states.

Nothing above should be construed to interfere with the sovereignty of the Departments of Health or Welfare or the Medical Societies of the individual compacting states.

HISTORY

Source. 1957, No. 154, § 1.

§ 705. Data; reports; research; fees—Article V

The board shall have the power to: collect, correlate, and evaluate data in the fields of its interest under this compact; to publish reports, bulletins and other documents making available the results of its research; and, in its discretion, to charge fees for said reports, bulletins and documents.

HISTORY

Source. 1957, No. 154, § 1.

§ 706. Gifts—Article VI

The board for the purposes of this compact is hereby empowered to receive grants, devises, gifts and bequests which the board may agree to accept and administer. The board shall administer property held in accordance with special trusts, grants and bequests, and shall also administer grants and devises of land and gifts or bequests of personal property made to the board for special uses, and shall execute said trusts, investing the proceeds thereof in notes or bonds secured by sufficient mortgages or other securities.

HISTORY

Source. 1957, No. 154, § 1.

212

§ 707. Separability of provisions—Article VII

The provisions of this compact shall be severable, and if any phrase, clause, sentence or provision of this compact is declared to be contrary to the constitution of any compacting state or of the United States the validity of the remainder of this compact and the applicability thereof to any government, agency, person or circumstance shall not be affected thereby; provided, that if this compact is held to be contrary to the constitution of any compacting state the compact shall remain in full force and effect as to all other compacting states.

HISTORY

Source. 1957, No. 154, § 1.

§ 708. Duration; withdrawal of membership—Article VIII

This compact shall continue in force and remain binding upon a compacting state until the legislature or the governor of such state, as the laws of such state shall provide, takes action to withdraw therefrom. Such action shall not be effective until two years after notice thereof has been sent by the governor of the state desiring to withdraw to the governors of the other states then parties to the compact. Such withdrawal shall not relieve the withdrawing state from its obligations accruing hereunder prior to the effective date of withdrawal. Any state so withdrawing, unless reinstated, shall cease to have any claim to or ownership of any of the property held by or vested in the board or to any of the funds of the board held under the terms of the compact. Thereafter, the withdrawing state may be reinstated by application after appropriate legislation is enacted by such state, upon approval by a majority of the board.

HISTORY

Source. 1957, No. 154, § 1.

§ 709. Default—Article IX

If any compacting state shall at any time default in the performance of any of its obligations assumed or imposed in accordance with the provisions of this compact, all rights and privileges and benefits conferred by this compact or agreement hereunder shall be suspended from the effective date of such default as fixed by the board. Unless such default shall be remedied within a period of two years following the effective date of such default, this compact may be terminated with respect to such defaulting state by affirmative vote of the other two member states. Any such defaulting state may be reinstated by (a) performing all acts and obligations upon which it has heretofore defaulted, and (b) application to and approval by a majority vote of the board.

HISTORY

Source. 1957, No. 154, § 1.

Subchapter 2. Provisions Relating to Compact

§ 741. Ratification

In order to provide advisory service to voluntary and official health agencies and educational institutions concerns with health, relating to policies concerned with the promotion, preservation and restoration of health and to insure the availability of day to day medical care where there is need in the rural areas of Maine, New Hampshire and Vermont.

The general assembly hereby ratifies the compact set out in subchapter 1 of this chapter to become effective at such time as the legislative bodies of the states of Maine and New Hampshire also ratify it.

HISTORY

Source. 1957, No. 154, § 1.

Revision note. Words "the following compact" were changed to "the compact set out in subchapter 1 of this chapter."

Adoption of compact. The Northern New England Medical Needs Compact was enacted by Maine Laws 1957, ch. 190, and New Hampshire Laws 1957, ch. 141.

§ 742. Copies

The secretary of state shall send authenticated copies of this chapter to the governor of each of the other two states party to this compact.

HISTORY

Source. 1957, No. 154, § 2.

§ 743. Exchange and filing of documents

The governor is authorized to take any action necessary to complete the exchange and filing of documents as between this state and any other state ratifying this compact.

HISTORY

Source. 1957, No. 154, § 3.

214

§ 744. Report

The members from this state shall obtain accurate accounts of all the board's receipts and disbursements and shall report to the governor on or before the fifteenth day of November, in even numbered years, the transactions of the board for the biennium ending on the preceding June thirtieth. They shall include in such report recommendations for any legislation which they consider necessary or desirable to carry out the intent and purposes of the compact.

HISTORY

Source. 1957, No. 154, § 4.

Appendix B

Congressional Testimony Outlining Rural Medical Needs—May 1958

STATEMENT OF DR. LEON R. LEZER, ASSOCIATE PROFESSOR OF PREVENTIVE MEDICINE AND DIRECTOR OF HEALTH STUDIES, COLLEGE OF MEDICINE, UNIVERSITY OF VERMONT

Dr. LEZER. Mr. Chairman and members of the Health and Science Subcommittee, I want to say first that I appreciate very much having the opportunity to appear here today. I would like to supplement some of the information that Congressman Coffin has already given you with respect to my own interests.

I am a rural person. I graduated from the University of Vermont College of Medicine. Up to now, I have had the opportunity to work in several phases of medical care, stemming from the general practice of medicine in a small rural community, to chief medical officer of the Presbyterian Hospital in Philadelphia, to assistant director of the Massachusettes General Hospital in Boston, and finally now, involved in medical education itself at the University of Vermont.

At our school, we are paying a great deal of attention to the factors which would promote interest on the part of future medical men in caring for populations such as we find in our rural areas, and I think successfully.

Being in touch with this rural problem, I would like to point out that our interests necessarily extend across the country. We have made it our business to learn to find out what is going on in rural medical care. So what I have to say does not confine itself by any means to Maine, New Hampshire, and Vermont. We have had many inquiries from across the country about our efforts in promoting available medical care to rural populations.

During the past 25 years American advancement in the medical sciences has made tremendous strides. Much has been accomplished by way of increasing life span, assuring survival of infants and preventing maternal deaths. Much has been accomplished to maintain the productivity of individuals and to promote the general health and welfare.

There are never advances of this magnitude without incidental creation of other problems. In the United States such problems have been produced which reflect most heavily in our rural areas. As medicine has advanced, it has become possible for the general physician to provide increasingly complex care to a large number of people. This factor has served to leave rural communities, which in the past had as many as 3 or 4 physicians, with none.

It is a certainty that the continuing loss of physicians in rural areas is not based on choice of residency in urban centers. I say this because we have discussed physician placement with so many young men looking for places to practice. We have had no difficulty, literally, in staffing some ten health centers which are the equivalent of the diagnostic treatment centers as intended by the Hill-Burton Act. The problem is one based on medical economics, both with respect to the consumer of medical care and the producer. With advances in medicine and with increasing skills the physician no longer finds it possible to practice medicine merely out of his black bag. Hence our approach, from two areas: (1) Medical education, and what are we expecting these men to do when they get out into practice; and (2) where can they practice the way they have been taught?

He must have available to him adequate facilities in order to maintain the high level of medical care for his patients as he understands it. After a long, expensive medical education, there are few physicians who find it possible to make the investment in facilities which would enable them to practice medicine according to competent standards. The laboratory is used routinely today in the practice of medicine just as the thermometer has been used routinely for many years.

The whole sequence of events has left rural areas unable to compete for services of physicians who might otherwise locate in rural areas. It is a well-known fact that our greatest problem in availability of medical services at the present time is not so much one of numbers of physicians as it is one of distribution of physicians. The choice of physicians in locating primarily in urban areas, where there are adequate facilities through community hospitals, relates directly to the problem of availability of physicians to rural areas.

It is important to the health of the Nation that rural areas be in a position to at least compete for physician services. It is an interesting fact that we are dealing with, not only a national problem, but an international phenomenon. Cities of the Eastern and the Western World have adequate availability of medical care. It is the villages and the less densely populated areas which have difficulty in maintaining the health of the people, and here in terms of our own strength in America, and in terms of our own productivity and advances on a proportionate basis with respect to availability of care in rural areas, we are not much different from India. Calcutta has excellent medical facilities. It is the villages and towns of India that have a problem.

We have the same problem, and this is why I choose to call it an international phenomenon. It is a well-known fact that the general level of health of those residing in urban centers is at a much higher plane than that of those residing in rural areas. The problem must be met by providing opportunity to rural areas to obtain day-to-day medical care in the form of suitable general practice facilities, and I say general practice facilities because I wish to reinforce what Dr. Hanley has already said: That 85 percent of the medical problems can be handled, and handled competently, by the general physician.

SCOPE OF THE PROBLEM

A unit of 2,500 or less has been considered to be a rural population. All communities coming under this definition of rural population have problems in availability of day-to-day medical care, and I mean literally all communities of this size in our country. The problem extends to those communities with populations amounting to 10,000 in many instances.

There is no one section of the country that has the matter of availability of medical care as a problem peculiarly its own. The tables attached will show a breakdown of the population problem as I am expressing it here, State by State, and on a community basis.

(The tables referred to are as follows:)

TABLE I.—*Population of the United States grouped according to counties by population of largest town in county*

[1950 census data]

	Number of counties [1]	Population	Percent of United States population	Cumulative population	Cumulative percent
Counties with no settlement of population greater than 1,000	330	2, 095, 107	1. 39	------------	---------
Counties the largest town of which is between 1,000 and 1,999	547	5, 986, 259	3. 97	8, 081, 366	5. 36
Counties the largest town of which is between 2,000 and 2,999	394	5, 975, 121	3. 96	14, 056, 487	9. 32
Counties the largest town of which is between 3,000 and 3,999	266	4, 751, 599	3. 15	18, 808, 086	12. 47
Counties the largest town of which is between 4,000 and 4,999	198	4, 310, 487	2. 86	23, 118, 573	15. 33
Counties the largest town of which is between 5,000 and 9,999	572	15, 628, 437	10. 37	38, 747, 010	25. 70
Counties whose largest town has a population greater than 10,000 (including the District of Columbia)	796	111, 950, 351	74. 29	150, 697, 361	99. 99
Total	3, 103	------------	---------	------------	---------

[1] Includes 3,070 counties, Baltimore City, St. Louis City, the District of Columbia, 27 independent cities in Virginia, and the parts of Yellowstone National Park in Idaho, Wyoming, and Montana.

TABLE II.—*Population by State, of all counties according to population of largest urban center in county, population of largest urban center*

[1950 census data]

State	Less than 1,000		1,000–1,999		2,000–2,999		3,000–3,999		4,000–4,999		5,000–9,999		10,000 plus, urban		Total	
	Number of counties	Population	Number of counties	Population	Number of counties	Population	Number of counties	Population	Number of counties	Population	Number of counties	Population	Number of counties	Population	Number of counties	Population
Alabama	3	58,240	11	212,368	8	180,337	9	224,910	3	84,106	18	633,686	15	1,668,096	67	3,061,743
Arizona			1	27,767			2	21,495	1	43,191	8	184,148	2	472,986	14	749,587
Arkansas	11	91,528	10	131,710	6	102,285	10	197,149	8	180,634	18	468,815	12	737,390	75	1,909,511
California	5	14,998	4	38,972	4	47,439	4	74,079	2	33,646	6	187,744	33	10,189,345	58	10,586,223
Colorado	14	31,166	16	77,609	7	60,387	3	27,553	4	45,903	10	225,619	9	856,852	63	1,325,089
Connecticut											1	44,709	7	1,962,571	8	2,007,280
Delaware											2	99,206	1	218,879	3	318,085
District of Columbia													1	802,178	1	802,178
Florida	5	17,578	10	60,183	12	130,289	5	69,588	7	87,021	7	190,442	21	2,216,204	67	2,771,305
Georgia	28	190,581	37	323,268	24	297,987	15	220,452	15	303,232	17	372,148	23	1,736,910	159	3,444,578
Idaho	[1] 9	20,572	10	61,088	6	44,446	4	38,192	6	80,683	2	37,900	8	305,756	[1] 45	588,637
Illinois	3	20,060	7	60,401	16	221,485	6	108,125	6	128,224	27	695,438	37	7,478,443	102	8,712,176
Indiana	2	15,498	7	70,980	11	163,280	7	166,688	4	77,565	30	670,706	31	2,769,507	92	3,934,224
Iowa			9	124,930	20	285,800	14	216,595	11	201,476	24	479,600	21	1,312,672	99	2,621,073
Kansas	7	27,177	29	191,510	21	183,161	8	92,591	7	100,908	10	220,157	23	1,089,795	105	1,905,299
Kentucky	21	185,949	38	504,514	11	157,122	11	218,116	8	158,741	17	539,601	14	1,180,763	120	2,944,806
Louisiana	3	25,246	11	155,161	6	114,310	7	149,012	7	148,338	14	424,186	16	1,667,083	64	2,683,516
Maine			1	18,004	1	18,617	2	52,787	1	35,187	5	229,853	6	559,326	16	913,774
Maryland	2	35,515	4	83,183	2	293,392	3	57,570	1	19,428	4	294,446	[2] 8	1,559,467	[2] 24	2,343,001
Massachusetts			1	5,633	1	3,484			1	46,805			11	4,634,592	14	4,690,514
Michigan	8	51,114	6	65,753	12	139,894	4	85,296	5	133,112	19	531,152	29	5,365,445	83	6,371,766
Minnesota	1	4,955	16	201,805	17	267,692	14	213,910	4	63,902	18	443,328	17	1,786,891	87	2,982,483
Mississippi	5	53,366	27	434,188	11	281,458	10	222,408	4	116,767	11	291,852	14	778,875	82	2,178,914
Missouri	13	105,379	32	352,940	14	194,959	10	163,868	9	182,950	18	450,631	[2] 19	2,503,926	[2] 115	3,954,653
Montana	[1] 14	37,093	15	67,837	9	85,532	6	51,203			6	93,547	7	255,812	[1] 57	591,024
Nebraska	19	54,479	28	209,629	13	114,354	10	136,068	4	47,198	9	136,871	10	626,911	93	1,325,510
Nevada	5	6,060	4	13,720	3	16,559	2	13,596			1	11,654	2	98,494	17	160,083
New Hampshire			1	15,868					1	47,923			8	469,451	10	533,242
New Jersey			3	187,849	1	164,371			1	42,736	3	143,261	13	4,297,112	21	4,835,329
New Mexico	1	3,533	8	85,199	2	14,144	2	23,387	3	39,337	9	156,891	7	358,696	32	681,187
New York	1	4,105	1	20,307	1	43,784	5	138,912	1	40,731	12	490,485	41	14,091,868	62	14,830,192
North Carolina	13	128,161	19	380,204	9	176,850	5	163,852	9	302,848	16	674,912	29	2,235,102	100	4,061,929
North Dakota	12	66,683	21	181,190	8	66,975			1	18,859	6	102,996	5	182,933	53	619,636
Ohio			5	68,991	9	203,133	3	67,861	4	96,552	19	561,520	48	6,948,570	88	7,946,627
Oklahoma	2	23,523	10	83,544	14	191,626	6	80,351	7	147,347	16	328,492	22	1,378,468	77	2,233,351
Oregon	4	14,449	4	25,912	1	6,649	5	67,758	3	72,507	9	354,514	10	979,552	36	1,521,341
Pennsylvania	2	11,689	3	34,055	2	41,548	5	119,490	2	73,818	13	587,450	40	9,629,962	67	10,498,012
Rhode Island											1	48,542	4	743,354	5	791,896

South Carolina	------	------	4	66,747	7	128,158	6	194,690	1	36,236	18	655,316	10	1,035,880	46	2,117,027
South Dakota	22	78,361	20	151,619	9	99,530	4	36,464	------	------	7	92,638	6	194,128	68	652,740
Tennessee	15	138,042	22	298,465	8	148,329	9	187,594	5	124,673	21	627,164	15	1,767,451	95	3,291,718
Texas	23	71,190	36	217,249	37	347,753	28	346,078	19	292,525	57	1,146,020	54	5,290,379	254	7,711,194
Utah	4	6,153	9	44,868	5	42,491	------	------	2	21,908	5	99,780	4	473,662	29	688,862
Vermont	1	.3,406	2	17,645	1	17,027	1	19,442	1	40,885	5	127,997	3	151,345	14	377,747
Virginia	38	401,270	16	272,220	17	458,345	6	203,095	8	267,608	[3] 18	386,779	[4] 24	1,329,363	[5] 127	3,318,680
Washington	4	15,964	6	55,532	2	11,444	2	47,711	2	40,904	6	146,781	17	2,060,627	39	2,378,963
West Virginia	5	60,280	12	158,102	9	182,101	2	54,724	4	164,830	11	409,099	12	976,416	55	2,005,552
Wisconsin	2	13,992	9	115,924	10	180,063	7	137,059	4	92,411	17	514,619	22	2,380,507	71	3,434,575
Wyoming	[1] 3	7,572	2	11,616	7	46,531	4	41,880	2	26,832	1	15,742	5	140,356	[1] 24	290,529
Total	------	2,095,107	------	5,986,259	------	5,975,121	------	4,751,599	------	4,310,487	------	15,628,437	------	111,950,351	------	150,697,361

[1] Includes part of Yellowstone National Park.
[2] Including 1 independent city.
[3] Including 7 independent cities.
[4] Including 20 independent cities.
[5] Including 27 independent cities.

Prepared by: A. F. Wessen, Ph. D.; K. B. Laughton, M. S.; University of Vermont, College of Medicine.

Prepared by A. F. Wessen, Ph. D., and K. B. Laughton, M. Sc., University of Vermont College of Medicine.

Table III.—*Percent population of States residing in counties by population of largest town in county*

[1950 census data]

State	Less than 1,000	1,000–1,999	2,000–2,999	3,000–3,999	4,000–4,999	5,000–9,999	10,000+
	Percent	Percent	Percent	Percent	Percent	Percent	Percent
Alabama	1.90	6.94	5.89	7.35	2.75	20.68	54.48
Arizona		3.70		2.87	5.76	24.57	63.10
Arkansas	4.79	6.90	5.36	10.32	9.46	24.55	38.62
California	.14	.37	.45	.70	.32	1.77	96.25
Colorado	2.35	5.86	4.56	2.08	3.46	17.03	64.66
Connecticut						2.23	97.77
Delaware						31.19	68.81
District of Columbia							100.00
Florida	.63	2.17	4.70	2.51	3.14	6.87	79.97
Georgia	5.53	9.38	8.65	6.40	8.80	10.81	50.43
Idaho	3.49	10.37	7.55	6.49	13.70	6.44	51.94
Illinois	.23	.69	2.54	1.24	1.47	7.98	85.84
Indiana	.39	1.80	4.15	4.24	1.97	17.05	70.40
Iowa		4.77	10.90	8.26	7.69	18.30	50.08
Kansas	1.43	10.05	9.61	4.86	5.30	11.55	57.20
Kentucky	6.31	17.13	5.34	7.41	5.39	18.32	40.10
Louisiana	.95	5.78	4.26	5.55	5.53	15.81	62.12
Maine		1.97	2.04	5.78	3.85	25.15	61.21
Maryland	1.52	3.55	12.52	2.46	.83	12.57	66.55
Massachusetts		.12	.07		1.00		98.81
Michigan	.80	1.03	2.20	1.34	2.09	8.34	84.20
Minnesota	.17	6.77	8.98	7.17	2.14	14.86	59.91
Mississippi	2.45	19.93	12.92	10.21	5.36	13.39	35.74
Missouri	2.66	8.92	4.93	4.14	4.63	11.39	63.32
Montana	6.28	11.48	14.47	8.66		15.83	43.28
Nebraska	4.11	15.81	8.63	10.27	3.56	10.33	47.29
Nevada	3.79	8.57	10.34	8.49		7.28	61.53
New Hampshire		2.97			8.99		88.04
New Jersey		3.88	3.40		.88	2.96	88.87
New Mexico	.52	12.51	2.08	3.43	5.77	23.03	52.66
New York	.03	.14	.29	.94	.27	3.31	95.02
North Carolina	3.15	9.36	4.35	4.03	7.46	16.62	55.03
North Dakota	10.76	29.24	10.81		3.04	16.62	29.52
Ohio		.87	2.56	.85	1.21	7.07	87.44
Oklahoma	1.05	3.74	8.58	3.60	6.60	14.71	61.72
Oregon	.95	1.70	.44	4.45	4.77	23.30	64.39
Pennsylvania	.11	.32	.40	1.14	.70	5.60	91.73
Rhode Island						6.13	93.87
South Carolina		3.15	6.05	9.20	1.71	30.95	48.93
South Dakota	12.00	23.23	15.25	5.59		14.19	29.74
Tennessee	4.19	9.07	4.51	5.70	3.79	19.05	53.69
Texas	.92	2.82	4.51	4.49	3.79	14.86	68.61
Utah	.89	6.51	6.17		3.18	14.48	68.76
Vermont	.90	4.67	4.51	5.15	10.82	33.88	40.07
Virginia	12.09	8.20	13.81	6.12	8.06	11.65	40.06
Washington	.67	2.33	.48	2.01	1.72	6.17	86.62
West Virginia	3.01	7.88	9.08	2.73	8.22	20.40	48.68
Wisconsin	.41	3.38	5.24	3.99	2.69	14.98	69.31
Wyoming	2.61	4.00	16.02	14.41	9.23	5.42	48.31
Total United States	1.39	3.97	3.96	3.15	2.86	10.37	74.29

Prepared by A. F. Wessen, Ph. D., and K. B. Laughton, M. Sc., University of Vermont College of Medicine.

Note.—Percentages are computed separately for each State.

Dr. Lezer. Table I, for example, shows the population of the United States grouped according to counties by population of the largest town in the county. Counties, the largest town of which is less than 3,000, account for 14,056,487 people. These are the communities across the country that have difficulty in maintaining daily availability of physician services. If we extend this figure to include counties, the largest town of which is less than 5,000, the problem is one which concerns more than 23 million people. In counties, the largest town of which is less than 10,000, we have a problem that is affecting nearly 39 million people.

Table II provides a breakdown of population in each State by largest urban center in a given county. Table III provides the same information but on a percentage basis.

Tables I, II, and III are a profile of the vast number of people who are in need of practicable assistance at the local level in order to compete for physician services.

The original Hill-Burton Hospital Construction Act did much to provide hospital facilities. It is now generally recognized, however, that a small hospital of 10 to 25 beds is neither an economically feasible unit nor a professionally sound operation. With the enactment of Public Law 482, 83d Congress, approved July 12, 1954, there came into being the opportunity to assist local rural areas with the problem of adequate facilities. It was the intent of this law that the diagnostic-treatment centers would materially assist in erasing inequities as to availability of medical care. The late Dr. John Cronin, the head of the Hospital Division, United States Public Health Service, discussed with me on several occasions the fact that the diagnostic-treatment center should be the facility that brought into action the line of medical services extending from the small rural area to the complex base hospital.

I would like to add here that in my contacts with the representatives of the American Hospital Association in Chicago, it is my impression that the American Hospital Association does enforce, in principle at least, the matter of a flow of services from the small community in the rural area to the hub where lies the base hospital. This is the concept.

Title VI of the Public Health Service Act, as amended, and issued in accordance with the requirements of Public Law 482, 83d Congress, states in Subpart H—Priority of Projects, section 53.71 (b) :

In determining the relative priority of projects, special consideration shall be given to those projects providing services to persons located in rural communities with relatively small financial resources.

Section 53.77 :

Diagnostic or treatment centers.—The priority of diagnostic or treatment center projects shall be determined after consideration of the following factors in the order of importance as given :

(a) The relative need for additional diagnostic or treatment services in the community or communities to be served by the project taking into account the existing or available services ;

(2) The extent to which diagnostic and treatment services will be made available to groups of the population which for any reason are less adequately served than other groups of the population.

The intent of Public Law 482, with respect to diagnostic treatment centers, therefore, is made clear. It is a fact that wherever there is in existence a community hospital, people will not be without medical care. People residing in urban centers or in communities that are sufficiently dense in population and have the economic resources to provide hospital facilities can always find medical care in these areas at any time of the day or night. The areas for which diagnostic-treatment centers were intended, as well as to provide expansion of outpatient-department services and diagnostic facilities to existing hospitals, are the areas referred to in tables I, II, and III.

After the initial experience of general hospital construction under the Hill-Burton Act, it became clear that we now live in an era of travel in time, not so much travel by miles. It is neither feasible nor professionally sound to try to have rural areas meet their daily medical-care problems by building more hospitals. The problem is one of providing a line of medical services as noted above and as so frequently stated to me by the late Dr. John Cronin.

Some things have been going on in our country. At the local level and on the voluntary part of people concerned, their own efforts, their own financial resources, a lot is going on, in spite of the fact that there is not available to these people funds which are in existence.

To one who is interested in problems of availability of medical care, it is readily apparent that small communities, such as represented in the attached tables, are doing everything within their own ability and resourcefulness to provide themselves with availability of physicians. Across the land small communities have done all manner of things in order to attract physicians. They have built homes; they have provided offices. Attempts to provide subsidy have failed, as have attempts to provide a bonus through tax resources at the local level.

Some 3 years ago a regional medical-needs committee was organized in northern New England as an advisory group to the University of Vermont College of Medicine, which had become very much interested in the problem of rural medical needs. This committee consisted of the officials of the three medical societies, the commissioners of health, and the deans of the Vermont and Dartmouth Medical Schools. At that time the regional medical-needs committee encouraged pursuit of problems in Public Law 482, which seemed to be barring rural areas from participating in already existing funds made available as grant-in-aid to meet local medical needs.

Since that time, the regional medical needs committee has become a regional medical needs board through appropriate legislation enacted in Maine, New Hampshire, and Vermont. The regional medical needs board has taken action, advising the University of Vermont College of Medicine, to work with the Sears-Roebuck Foundation in assisting with provision of health centers or diagnostic-treatment centers in small rural areas in order that there may be opportunity for these people to compete with urban centers for the availability of physicians. The Sears-Roebuck Foundation is doing much across the country to assist areas in establishing facilities to attract physicians. I would like to point out that the Sears-Roebuck Foundation operates its program under endorsement of the American Medical Association. I would like also to point out that the efforts of a private foundation do not take the place of public responsibility, but rather complement it, it seems to me, in our form of government.

The American Medical Association has published a pamphlet entitled "How a Community Gets Its Doctor." This pamphlet carries the name of the Chelsea Health Center in Chelsea, Vt., as one effort which succeeded along these lines. The Chelsea Health Center is a nonprofit corporation established by the private resources of local people in five small rural communities. It is in effect the type of facility intended in the diagnostic-treatment center provisions of Public Law 482.

The problem is being met in northern New England through the formation of nonprofit corporations at the local level. People in small rural communities are raising funds the hard way in order to provide themselves with the equivalent of a diagnostic-treatment center in order to attract physicians. Some 10 of these centers have met with outstanding success in recruiting physicians. This they must do because funds which would otherwise be available through already existing Federal tax resources have not reached them.

I wish, gentlemen, it were possible for you to get the picture I have in working in these small rural areas, seeing these local folks—the postman, the selectman, the housewife, the farmer, the local store-owners—pooling their own resources and their own ingenuity and effort in order to provide themselves with day-to-day medical care.

PROBLEM WITH PUBLIC LAW

Public Law 482, which provided for diagnostic-treatment centers, has effectively, although unintentionally, barred rural areas from taking advantage of tax funds. It has been established that only two health centers have been built in rural areas since the original passage of this law. The problem lies in restriction as to applicant.

Congressman Coffin has very ably pointed out in the Congressional Record of the House, dated April 2, 1958, the difficulties as to eligibility for application with this restriction in rural areas. In the Congressional Record of the Senate dated June 11, 1956, Senator Flanders pointed out similar problems as to rural areas with the restriction in application.

With the provision for formal affiliation with a nonprofit teaching hospital, the protection of hospital interest in the sale of their services is assured. Even more important, it assures a high quality of medical care at the rural level.

I would like to point out here that there is nothing cumbersome or difficult about a formal affiliation with a nonprofit teaching hospital. As a matter of fact, we have much of this going on already but not on a formal, organized basis. We do have physicians who travel out to rural areas to some extent in consultation. We do have physicians from rural areas who go to the metropolitan areas in order to maintain their professional growth. There is some of this already.

In our own area we have had a great deal of direct assistance from the teaching hospital, in the form of providing technical assistance, training, laboratory aids, and the like.

There is no difference between a physician renting space and facilities in a nonprofit corporation at the rural level and in a physician renting an office in a hospital. Many physicians rent offices in hospitals or in other professional facilities, and there is more and more of that going on.

ACCOMPLISHMENT BY AMENDING PUBLIC LAW 482 AS SUGGESTED IN
H. R. 11826

If the 85th Congress in its 2d session sees fit to amend Public Law 482, title VI of the Public Health Service Act, it will have done much to make it possible for rural areas to provide themselves with adequate availability of day-to-day medical care. It will have made it possible for physicians to practice in rural areas who otherwise, frequently because of medical economics, will seek out urban centers where they will have at their disposal hospital services, thereby avoiding heavy investment in facilities which they can ill afford in most instances after a long, expensive medical education.

The administration of this section of the act as suggested for amendment in H. R. 11826 does not change the basic requirements of approval through a sole State agency which in most instances is the State health department. The requirement that there be shown an actual affiliation with a nonprofit teaching hospital provides protection for hospitals as noted above, as well as an increase in the level of quality of medical care in the rural area.

We are a mighty nation and we should not have common to us problems in adequacy of rural medical care which exists in many so-called underprivileged countries of the world. Proportionate to our rate of growth and strength that lie in America, we do not present the healthy picture for our rural areas that we should present in our position of international leadership. Amending title VI of the Public Health Service Act as suggested in H. R. 11826, will do much to correct inequities in availability of medical services, to improve distribution of physicians, and to increase preventive services which come first and foremost in maintaining the health of a nation.

Gentlemen, I thank you, and I shall be very happy to answer any questions that you desire to ask.

Mr. O'Brien. Doctor, I just want to say it is a pleasure to have you here. I know in my community we have several fine physicians who are graduates of the University of Vermont.

Do you believe that the adoption of the amendment proposed by Congressman Coffin will in effect carry out the original intent of Public Law 482?

Dr. Lezer. Yes, sir; I do.

Mr. O'Brien. That the Congress intended in 482 to do what you now propose?

Dr. Lezer. Yes, sir.

Mr. O'Brien. But somewhere along the line, in the chain of command, things got garbled? Is that what you are saying?

Dr. Lezer. Yes. We have, Mr. Chairman, consulted with a number of hospitals, asking:

Under the present law would you apply for funds in order to establish a diagnostic-treatment facility in Town X, which is 40 miles away?

In each instance, the answer is:

No; we will not become legally or financially involved in a unit that is 30 or 40 miles away.

Proposal No. 2:

If this law were amended in order that you could support and assist such a center but not be involved legally or financially, would you support and assist it?

The answer to this has been invariably "Yes," or "we would certainly bring this up with our board of trustees."

Mr. O'Brien. Thank you, Doctor.

Mr. Loser?

Mr. LOSER. I would say that the distinguished doctor is a magnificent advocate of the cause he espouses.

Dr. LEZER. Thank you.

Mr. O'BRIEN. Mr. Bush?

Mr. BUSH. I want to thank the doctor for a very fine presentation. It has been very informative, and will be a great contribution to the committee.

Mr. O'BRIEN. Dr. Neal?

Mr. NEAL. I recognize the doctor's testimony here as coming from a man who knows the problem from the ground up.

Dr. LEZER. Thank you, sir.

Mr. NEAL. I was wondering, Doctor. Most of the larger hospitals in congested areas maintain closed staffs?

Dr. LEZER. That is right, sir.

Mr. NEAL. Do you feel that if these hospitals maintained a more liberal practice toward the men out in the field who are general practitioners, gave them a little bit more liberty, made them a little more welcome, in some of these larger closed-staff hospitals, it would help to solve the problem to some extent?

Dr. LEZER. I think it would help tremendously from the standpoint of the physicians' continuing professional growth. I do not think, Dr. Neal, that it would materially assist in these areas which do not have the density of population or the economic resources to challenge a physician in a specialty practice. And the areas that we are talking about are these groups of communities several of which make up, say, 3,000 or 4,000 people. I do not think the open staff of the teaching hospital would help that. But it would help the physician who was in those areas.

We are encouraging open staff, and both our hospitals connected with the medical school do have open staff. We have a general practice division in the medical school with general physicians on the faculty. But this kind of thing, I think, is extremely important, as an associated problem with this.

Mr. NEAL. Thank you, Doctor. Your testimony has been very interesting and quite helpful.

Dr. LEZER. Thank you very much.

Mr. O'BRIEN. Thank you, Doctor.

Appendix C

Resolution of a State Legislature Enlisting Consultation of a State Medical School's Department of Community Medicine—1959

NO. R-63—JOINT RESOLUTION RELATING TO INTERIM COMMISSION ON TUBERCULOSIS.

Whereas, it appears that tuberculosis in Vermont may continue to be a major health problem for some years to come, despite a decrease in the number of new cases and in deaths thereform in recent years, and

Whereas, advances in the treatment of tuberculosis in recent years tend towards the possibility of eradication or of minimizing the incidence of this disease, and

Whereas, both from a standpoint of health and of the alleviation of a drain upon the economic resources of the state, it appears desirable that Vermont should make a concerted effort to eradicate tuberculosis and to that end should formulate an up-to-date program based upon a study of the problem in the light of new developments, particularly in the fields of information, case findings and treatment, and

Whereas, the department of preventive medicine of the University of Vermont college of Medicine in conjunction with the

Vermont tuberculosis and health association completed a study of tuberculosis control in Vermont, which report is dated February, 1959, now therefore be it

Resolved by the Senate and House of Representatives:

That the department of preventive medicine of the University of Vermont College of Medicine in cooperation with the department of health and the Vermont tuberculosis association, be requested to submit to the 1961 Legislature findings and recommendations for a program to eradicate tuberculosis in Vermont.

Approved: June 11, 1959.

Notes

Part I

[1]Bean, W. B., *Journal of the American Medical Association*, 154:639, February 20, 1954.

[2]Wells, R. Lomax, "Medical Examinations in Industry," *A.M.A. Archives of Industrial Health*, 14:6, pp. 503–509, December 1956.

[3]Kelly, E. Lowell, "Multiple Criteria of Medical Education and Their Applications for Selection: The Appraisal of Applicants to Medical Schools," A Report of the Fourth Teaching Institute, Association of American Medical Colleges, 1957.

[4]Berry, George Packer, "Medical Education in Transition," *Journal of Medical Education*, vol. 20, no. 3, March 1953.

[5]Lezer, Leon R. "An Experimental Approach to the Teaching of Human Ecology," *Journal of Medical Education*, vol. 34, no. 6, pp. 593–600, June 1959.

[6]Rosen, George, A *History of Public Health*, Publications, Inc., New York, 1958.

[7]Smillie, Wilson G., *Public Health: Its Promise for the Future*, Macmillan Company, New York, 1955.

[8]Stocking, Fred H., "The Important Balance," Harvard Graduate School of Education Association, vol. 4, no. 3, Special Edition, 1959.

[9]Curran, Jean A., and Cockerill, Eleanor, "Widening Horizons in Medical Education," *Joint Committee on the Teaching of Social and Environmental Factors in Medicine*, Harvard University Press, 1948.

[10]Robinson, G. Canby, "The Study of the Patient as a Whole as Training for Medical Practice," *Journal of the Association of American Medical Colleges*, 14:65, March 1939.

[11]Robinson, G. Canby, "The Patient As A Person: A Study of the Social Aspects of Illness," The Commonwealth Fund, New York, New York, 1939.

[12]Leavell, Hugh and Clark, E. Gurney, et.al., *Preventive Medicine for the Doctor in His Community: A Epidemiologic Approach*, 3rd. Ed., McGraw-Hill, New York, 1965.

[13]Darley, W., "Medical Education, Specialty Practice and the Family Doctor," *Rocky Mountain Medical Journal*, 49:35–40, 1952.

[14]Trussell, Ray E., *Hunterdon Medical Center: The Story of One Approach to Rural Medical Care*, Harvard University Press, 1956.

[15]Leavell, Hugh R. and Clark, E. Gurney et.al, *Preventive Medicine for the Doctor in His Community: An Epidemiologic Approach*, 3rd Ed., McGraw-Hill, New York, 1965.

Part II

[1]Trussell, Ray E., *Hunterdon Medical Center: The Story of One Approach to Rural Medical Care*, Harvard University Press, 1956.

[2]Rosenfeld, L. S. and Makover, H. B., *The Rochester Regional Hospital Council*, Harvard University Press, 1956.

[3]Selwyn-Brown, Arthur, *The Physician Throughout the Ages*, Vol. II, Capehart-Brown Co., New York, N.Y. 1928.

[4]Smillie, Wilson G., *Public Health: Its Promise for the Future*, The Macmillan Co., New York, N.Y., 1955.

[5]McIntire, Charles: "The Importance of the Study of Medical Sociology," *Bulletin of the American Academy of Medicine* (now *Journal of Sociological Medicine*), I, pp. 425–434, 1894.

[6]Orr, Louis M., "The President's Page," *Journal of the American Medical Association*, Vol. 172, No. 9, 945, February 27, 1960.

[7]Porterfield, Austin L., "Social Knowledge in Medicine," *Journal of Health and Human Behavior*, Vol. 1, No. 1, 1960.

[8]Rosen, George, History, "Sociology and Innovation in the Provision of Medical Care," Paper presented to the Medical Care Section, 86th Annual Meeting, the American Public Health Association, St. Louis, Mo., October 29, 1958.

[9]Selwyn-Brown, Arthur, *The Physician Throughout the Ages*, Vol. 1, pp. 88-89, 96, Capehart-Brown Co., Inc. New York, New York, 1928.

[10]Ibid.

[11]Rosen, George, Op. cit.

[12]Goldman, Franz, *Public Medical Care*, Columbia University Press, New York, 1945.